ATLAS *of* RETINAL **OCT**

OPTICAL COHERENCE TOMOGRAPHY

Second Edition

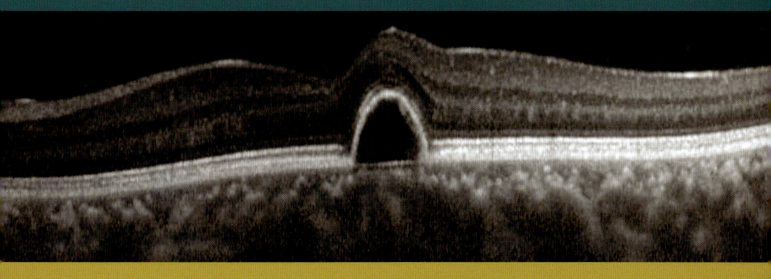

ATLAS *of* RETINAL OCT
OPTICAL COHERENCE TOMOGRAPHY

Shilpa J. Desai, MD
Assistant Professor
Director, Medical Student Education
Director, Retinopathy of Prematurity Service
Vitreoretinal Surgery and Ocular Oncology
Department of Ophthalmology
New England Eye Center
Tufts Medical Center
Tufts University School of Medicine
Boston, MA
United States

Darin R. Goldman, MD
Partner, Retina Group of Florida
Clinical Affiliate Associate Professor of Surgery
Charles E Schmidt College of Medicine
Florida Atlantic University
Boca Raton, FL
United States

Nadia K. Waheed, MD, MPH
Professor
Ophthalmology
New England Eye Center
Tufts Medical Center
Tufts University School of Medicine
Boston, MA
United States

Jay S. Duker, MD
Professor
Department of Ophthalmology
New England Eye Center
Tufts Medical Center
Tufts University School of Medicine
Boston, MA
United States

ELSEVIER

Elsevier
1600 John F. Kennedy Blvd.
Ste 1800
Philadelphia, PA 19103-2899

ATLAS OF RETINAL OCT: OPTICAL COHERENCE TOMOGRAPHY, SECOND EDITION

ISBN: 978-0-323-93043-7

Notice

Practitioners and researchers must always rely on their own experience and knowledge in evaluating and using any information, methods, compounds, or experiments described herein. Because of rapid advances in the medical sciences in particular, independent verification of diagnoses and drug dosages should be made. To the fullest extent of the law, no responsibility is assumed by Elsevier, authors, editors, or contributors for any injury and/or damage to persons or property as a matter of products liability, negligence, or otherwise, or from any use or operation of any methods, products, instructions, or ideas contained in the material herein.

Previous edition copyrighted 2018

Senior Content Development Manager: Somodatta Roy Choudhury
Senior Content Strategist: Kayla Wolfe
Senior Content Development Specialist: Vasowati Shome
Publishing Services Manager: Shereen Jameel
Project Manager: Vishnu T. Jiji
Senior Designer: Brian Salisbury

Printed in India

Last digit is the print number: 9 8 7 6 5 4 3 2 1

Working together
to grow libraries in
developing countries

www.elsevier.com • www.bookaid.org

To my wonderful parents, whom I can never thank enough. And to my husband and three children—you are a source of strength, joy, and inspiration to me each day.

S.J.D.

To my wife Robin for her unwavering love and support, and to my children, Rona, Cole, and Lexi, who add immeasurable joy and fulfillment to our lives.

D.R.G.

To Jujie, Memsie, and Ammi, without whom none of this would have been possible.

N.K.W.

To my colleagues at the New England Eye Center who have assisted me in bringing innovation to eye care for over three decades.

J.S.D.

Contributors

OMAR ABU-QAMAR, MD, MMSC
Resident Physician, Ophthalmology
New England Eye Center
Tufts Medical Center
Tufts University School of Medicine
Boston, MA
United States

A. YASIN ALIBHAI, MD
Director
Boston Image Reading Center
Boston, MA
United States

CAROLINE R. BAUMAL, MD
Professor of Ophthalmology
New England Eye Center
Tufts Medical Center
Tufts University School of Medicine
Boston, MA
United States

JONATHAN T. CARANFA, MD, PHARMD
Physician Resident, Ophthalmology
New England Eye Center
Tufts Medical Center
Tufts University School of Medicine
Boston, MA
United States

YI LING DAI, MD
Ophthalmologist
New England Eye Center
Tufts Medical Center
Tufts University School of Medicine
Boston, MA
United States

SHILPA J. DESAI, MD
Assistant Professor
Director, Medical Student Education
Director, Retinopathy of Prematurity Service
Vitreoretinal Surgery and Ocular Oncology
Department of Ophthalmology
New England Eye Center
Tufts Medical Center
Tufts University School of Medicine
Boston, MA
United States

IVANA N. DESPOTOVIC, MD
Neuro-Ophthalmologist
Boston Image Reading Center
St. Louis, MA
United States

DARIN R. GOLDMAN, MD
Partner, Retina Group of Florida
Clinical Affiliate Associate Professor of Surgery
Charles E Schmidt College of Medicine
Florida Atlantic University
Boca Raton, FL
United States

CHELSEA GOTTSCHALK, MD
Comprehensive Ophthalmology
Lexington Eye Associates
Lexington, MA
United States

MATTHEW N. HENDERSON, BA
MD Candidate, Class of 2023
Rutgers Robert Wood Johnson Medical School
New Brunswick, NJ
United States

KATE V. HUGHES, MD
Resident Physician, Ophthalmology
New England Eye Center
Tufts Medical Center
Tufts University School of Medicine
Boston, MA
United States

ERIN M. LANZO, MA, MD
Ophthalmology Resident
New England Eye Center
Tufts Medical Center
Tufts University School of Medicine
Boston, MA
United States

JOAO VICTOR PERES LIMA, MD, ICBS, UFMA
Ophthalmologist
Universidade Federal do Pará
Belem, Para;
Retina Fellowship
HOPR
Parana, Parana
Brazil

PHOEBE L. MELLEN, MD
Fellow, Retina
New England Eye Center
Tufts Medical Center
Tufts University School of Medicine
Boston, MA
United States

NORA W. MUAKKASSA, MD
Clinical Associate
Ophthalmology
New England Eye Center
Tufts Medical Center
Tufts University School of Medicine
Boston, MA
United States

TAVISH NANDA, MD
Ophthalmologist
New England Eye Center
Tufts Medical Center
Tufts University School of Medicine
Boston, MA
United States

CARLOS A. MOREIRA NETO, MD, PHD, MSC
Director, Retina
Hospital de Olhos do Paraná
Curitiba
Brazil

EDUARDO A. NOVAIS, MD
Collaborator, Ophthalmology
Federal University of São Paulo
São Paulo, SP
Brazil

ALLISON RESNIK, MD
Resident Physician, Ophthalmology
New England Eye Center
Tufts Medical Center
Tufts University School of Medicine
Boston, MA
United States

LUIZ ROISMAN, MD, PHD
Ophthalmologist
Universidade do Estado do Rio de Janeiro
Rio de Janeiro
Brazil

ANGELL SHI, MD
Resident Physician, Ophthalmology
New England Eye Center
Tufts Medical Center
Tufts University School of Medicine
Boston, MA
United States

EDUARDO UCHIYAMA, MD
Uveitis Specialist/Vitreo-Retinal Surgeon
Retina Group of Florida
Fort Lauderdale, FL;
Affiliate Assistant Professor
Charles E. Schmidt College of Medicine
Florida Atlantic University
Boca Raton, FL
United States

NADIA K. WAHEED, MD, MPH
Professor
Ophthalmology
New England Eye Center
Tufts Medical Center
Tufts University School of Medicine
Boston, MA
United States

ANTONIO YAGHY, MD
Researcher, Oncology
Wills Eye Hospital
Philadelphia, PA
United States

JAY S. DUKER, MD
Professor
Department of Ophthalmology
New England Eye Center
Tufts Medical Center
Tufts University School of Medicine
Boston, MA
United States

DANIELA FERRARA, MD, PHD, FASRS
Assistant Professor of Ophthalmology
New England Eye Center
Tufts Medical Center
Tufts University School of Medicine
Boston, MA
United States

Preface

Optical coherence tomography (OCT) continues to grow and expand its reach within ophthalmology. OCT is now widely available and has become a prerequisite part of the comprehensive ophthalmic exam, especially in retina. Although a relatively recent technology, OCT findings have now become critical to making certain diagnoses. Alterations in each layer of the retina differentiate between pathologies and explain visual changes.

The second edition of the *Atlas of Retinal OCT* is a continuation of the first edition with the addition of new pathologies and OCT angiography where applicable. This atlas is meant to serve as a reference for a breadth of retinal conditions—from those seen in everyday practice to more rare and unique pathologies. Each condition is illustrated with numerous, large, high-quality OCT images to highlight disease pathology and aid in disease identification. Additional imaging modalities, such as fundus photographs and fluorescein angiograms, are included to supplement OCT images where appropriate.

Atlas of Retinal OCT provides the reader with a high-quality, easy-to-follow visual aid to help incorporate OCT scans into the evaluation and care of your patients. The atlas is designed to make OCT more comprehensible for both the novice and expert clinician. We hope you find this to be a handy and practical addition to your everyday references.

Acknowledgments

A project such as this requires contributions from many different groups and individuals to be successful. First and foremost, the images used in this atlas would not be possible without our many patients. We are very grateful to these individuals who trust their care in our hands on a daily basis. Additionally, we rely on the talented photographers and technical staff at both New England Eye Center at Tufts Medical Center and the Retina Group of Florida to obtain the majority of the included OCT images. Their expertise is reflected in the volume of high-quality images available for inclusion in this project. We would also like to thank the many coauthors who have contributed to various chapters throughout the atlas. Lastly, the professionalism and expertise of the staff at Elsevier are unmatched. We want to thank the entire team at Elsevier who were critical to the completion of this project, in particular Vasowati Shome and Kayla Wolfe.

Contents

Normal Optic Nerve   1.1

Carlos A. Moreira Neto

Summary

Spectral domain (SD) OCT devices have two scan patterns used to analyze the optic nerve head: volume scans and line scans.

Volume Scans

Volume scans acquire a volumetric set of data, centered at the optic nerve head. It delineates the optic disc margin and optic disc surface contour and is segmented to obtain the retinal nerve fiber boundaries. Each device has its own scanning protocol. The Cirrus HD-OCT identifies the center of the optic disc and creates a 3.46 mm circle on this location and calculates the thickness of the retinal nerve fiber layer (RNFL). The Heidelberg Spectralis creates a cylindrical volume with a diameter of 3.4 mm through and around the optic nerve head (Duker et al., 2014). The Optovue RTVue's protocol for the optic nerve head consists of a grid pattern with circular and radial scans that acquires a 4 mm × 4 mm volume around the optic nerve. Because different machines use circles of different diameters around the center of the optic nerve head, the measurement of RNFL between machines is not comparable (Duker et al., 2014).

Retinal Nerve Fiber Layer Thickness

OCT devices calculate RNFL thickness as the distance between the internal limiting membrane and the outer aspect of the RNFL (Fig. 1.1.1).

Ganglion Cell Complex

The ganglion cell complex (GCC) consists of the thickness of three inner retinal layers: the nerve fiber layer (NFL), the ganglion cell layer, and the inner plexiform layer. The scan must be centered at the fovea, and the software presents the results as color-coded "map," compared to a normative database (Fig. 1.1.2).

Optic Nerve Morphology

SD-OCT devices also calculate optic nerve diameter, area, cup, and rim measurements (Fig. 1.1.1). Each measurement varies according to age (Cavallotti et al., 2002) and ethnicity (Girkin, 2008). According to Budenz et al., the mean RNFL thickness in a normal population is 100.1 µm. Thinner RNFL measurements were associated with older age. Caucasians had slightly thinner RNFL than Hispanics or Asians. People with smaller optic disc area also have thinner RNFL (Budenz et al., 2007).

Line Scans

Aiming to obtain a higher-resolution visualization of structure and anatomical anomalies at the optic nerve head, line scans provide a single or a series of high-resolution B-scans similar to the scans obtained in the macula (Fig. 1.1.3).

OCTA has given a greater insight into optic disc vasculature and peripapillary vessel density, which could help to have a better understanding of the role of this vascular bed in the functioning of the RNFL (Fig. 1.1.4).

REFERENCES

Budenz, D. L., Anderson, D. R., Varma, R., Schuman, J., Canotr, L., Savell, J. et al. (2007). Determinants of normal retinal nerve fiber layer thickness measured by Stratus OCT. *Ophthalmology, 114*(6), 1046–1052.

Cavallotti, C., Pacella, E., Pescosolido, N., Tranquilli-Leali, F. M., & Feher, J. (2002). Age-related changes in the human optic nerve. *Canadian Journal of Ophthalmology, 37*(7), 389–394.

Duker, J. S., Waheed, N. K., & Goldman, D. R. (2014). Scanning principles. *Handbook of retinal OCT*. St. Louis: Elsevier.

Girkin, C. A. (2008). Differences in optic nerve structure between individuals of predominantly African and European ancestry: Implications for disease detection and pathogenesis. *Clinical Ophthalmology, 2*(1), 65–69.

ONH and RNFL OU Analysis: Optic Disc Cube 200×200 OD ● | ○ OS

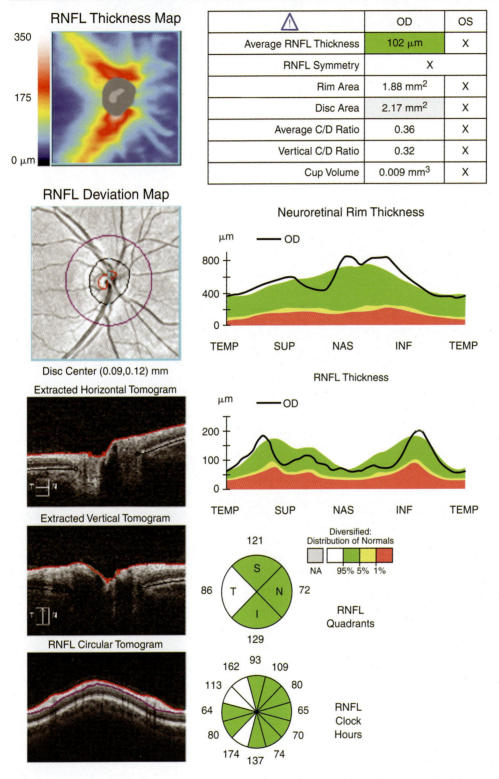

RNFL Thickness Map

350

175

0 μm

⚠	OD	OS
Average RNFL Thickness	102 μm	X
RNFL Symmetry	X	
Rim Area	1.88 mm²	X
Disc Area	2.17 mm²	X
Average C/D Ratio	0.36	X
Vertical C/D Ratio	0.32	X
Cup Volume	0.009 mm³	X

RNFL Deviation Map

Disc Center (0.09,0.12) mm

Extracted Horizontal Tomogram

Extracted Vertical Tomogram

RNFL Circular Tomogram

Neuroretinal Rim Thickness

μm ── OD

800

400

0

TEMP SUP NAS INF TEMP

RNFL Thickness

μm ── OD

200

100

0

TEMP SUP NAS INF TEMP

Diversified:
Distribution of Normals

NA 95% 5% 1%

121
S
86 T N 72
I
129

RNFL
Quadrants

93
162   109
113   80
64   65
80   70
174 137 74

RNFL
Clock
Hours

FIG. 1.1.1 Peripapillary RNFL and neuro-retinal rim thickness and disc area measurements using a SD-OCT, in a normal patient. *INF*, inferior; *NAS*, nasal; *OD*, Right eye; *ONH*, Optic nerve head; *OS*, left eye; *RNFL*, retinal nerve fiber layer; *SD*, spectral domain; *SUP*, superior; *TEMP*, temporal. (Courtesy of Carlos A. Moreira Neto.)

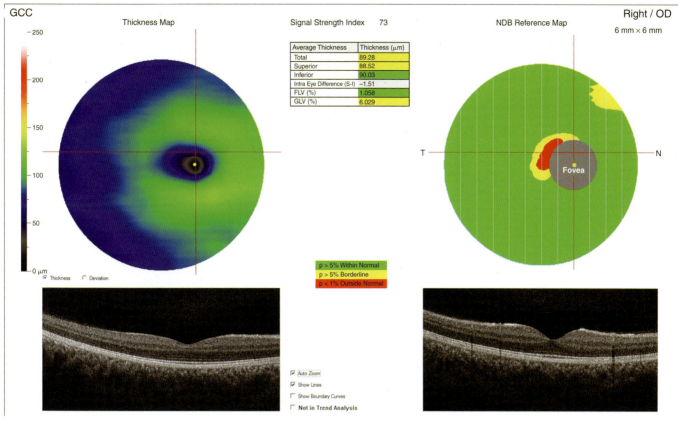

GCC

Thickness Map

Signal Strength Index   73

NDB Reference Map

Right / OD

6 mm × 6 mm

Average Thickness	Thickness (μm)
Total	89.28
Superior	88.52
Inferior	90.03
Intra Eye Difference (S-I)	−1.51
FLV (%)	1.058
GLV (%)	6.029

- p > 5% Within Normal
- p > 5% Borderline
- p < 1% Outside Normal

○ Thickness   ○ Deviation

Fovea

T   N

☑ Auto Zoom
☑ Show Lines
☐ Show Boundary Curves
☐ Not in Trend Analysis

FIG. 1.1.2 Color-coded ganglion cell complex thickness using a spectral domain OCT, in a normal patient. *FLV*, Focal loss volume; *GLV*, global loss volume; *NDB*, Normative database; *OD*, right eye. (Courtesy of Carlos A. Moreira Neto.)

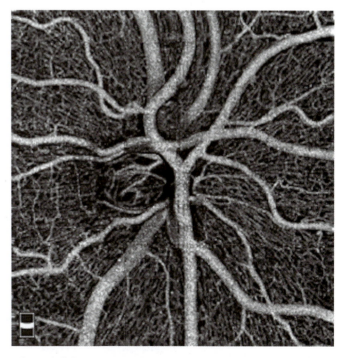

FIG. 1.1.3 Line scan of the optic nerve head. (Courtesy of Carlos A. Moreira Neto.)

FIG. 1.1.4 OCT angiography (3 mm × 3 mm) of the optic nerve head. (Courtesy of Carlos A. Moreira Neto.)

Time Domain OCT

Carlos A. Moreira Neto

2.1

Summary

The first OCT image, published by Huang et al. (1991), was captured using a device that detected light echoes using time domain detection. In time domain (TD)-OCT, the reference arm, with a physically moving mirror, and a sample arm undergo interference, which is used to generate an A-scan. Multiple A-scans obtained linearly are combined to generate a cross-sectional B-scan) (Duker et al., 2014). (Fig. 2.1.1)

REFERENCES

Duker, J. S., Waheed, N. K., & Goldman, D. R. (2014). Scanning principles. *Handbook of retinal OCT*. St. Louis: Elsevier.
Huang, D., Swanson, E. A., Lin, C. P., Schuman, J. S., Stinson, W. G., Change, W., et al. (1991). Optical coherence tomography. *Science, 254*(5035), 1178–1181.

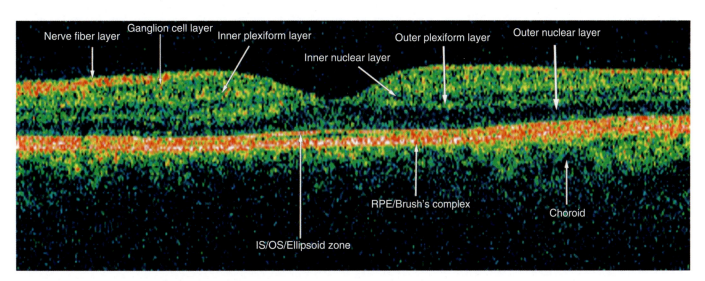

FIG. 2.1.1 Normal macula imaged using time domain OCT. *IS/OS/EZ*, Inner segment/outer segment/ellipsoid zone; *RPE*, retinal pigment epithelium. (Courtesy Dr. Jayme Arana, Hospital de Olhos do Paraná.)

Summary

In spectral domain (SD) OCT, a spectral interference pattern between the reference beam and the sample beam is obtained simultaneously by a spectrometer and an array detector. Unlike time domain (TD) OCT, SD-OCT does not require a physically moving reference mirror, instead using frequency information to produce interference patterns. This allows for much faster acquisition and higher-quality images than TD-OCT.

The high resolution provided by SD-OCT allows for the visualization of the microscopic anatomy of the retina (Fig. 2.2.1) with more details than TD-OCT images.

Because the retinal pigment epithelium (RPE) is highly hyper-reflective with OCT imaging, there is a limited penetration of light beyond it, decreasing the resolution of the choroid (Joel Schuman et al., 2013). Normal mean central foveal thickness is 225.1 ± 17.1 µm, as measured by SD-OCT, although this varies with age and retinal status.

REFERENCE

Joel Schuman, C. P., Fujimoto, J., & Duker, J. (2013). *Optical coherence tomography of ocular diseases*. 3rd ed. Thorofare, NJ: Slack Incorporated.

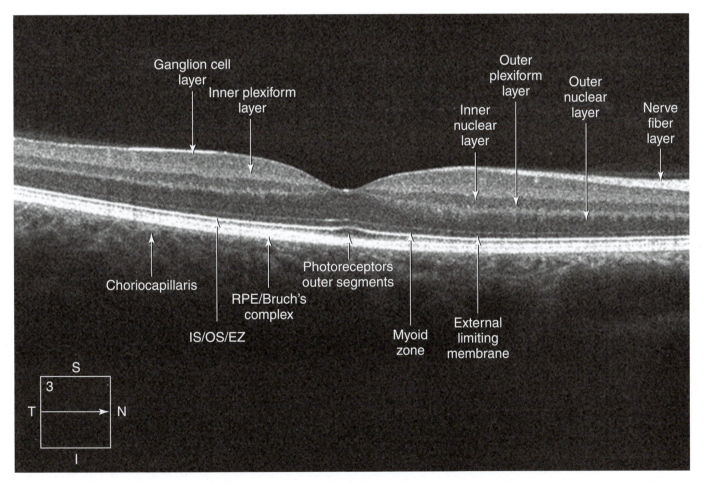

FIG. 2.2.1 Normal macula imaged using spectral domain OCT. *IS/OS/EZ*, Inner segment/outer segment/ellipsoid zone; *RPE*, retinal pigment epithelium.

Summary

Swept source (SS) OCT is a modified Fourier-domain and depth resolved technology that offers potential advantages over spectral domain (SD) OCT, including reduced sensitivity roll-off with imaging depth, higher detection efficiencies, improved imaging range, and better penetration of the choroid (Fig. 2.3.1). In SS-OCT, a narrow-band light source is rapidly swept through a wide range of frequencies. The interference pattern is detected on a single or small number of receivers as a function of time.

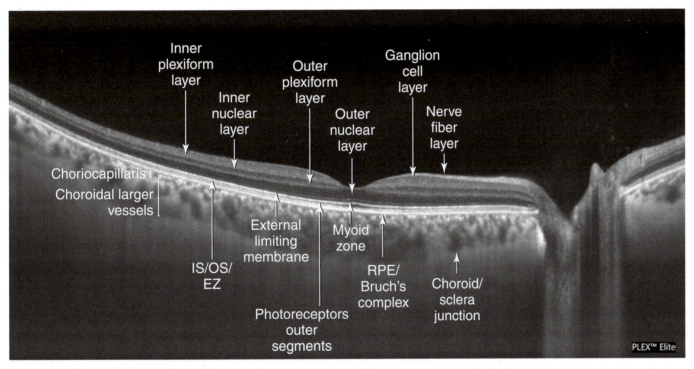

FIG. 2.3.1 Normal retina imaged using swept source OCT. *EZ*, Ellipsoid zone; *IS*, inner segments; *OS*, outer segments; *RPE*, retinal pigment epithelium.

Normal Choroid | 3.1

Carlos A. Moreira Neto

Summary

Enhanced depth imaging (EDI) on commercially available OCT devices allows for higher-quality images of the choroid (Fig. 3.1.1). EDI mode moves the zero-delay line of the spectral domain (SD) OCT closer to the choroid, enabling better visualization of choroidal structures and a more precise measurement of choroidal thickness than standard OCT scanning protocols. This is useful for diseases, such as central serous chorioretinopathy, in which the choroidal-scleral interface may be difficult to visualize. Studies of choroidal thickness in normal subjects and those with pathology have shown a wide variation in measurements (Fujiwara et al., 2012; Margolis & Spaide, 2009).

The choroid is divided into three layers, the choriocapillaris or smaller blood vessels, the Sattler's layer, and the Haller's layer or larger blood vessels (Fig. 3.1.2).

REFERENCES

Fujiwara, A., Shiragami, C., Shirakata, Y., Manabe, S., Izumibata, S., & Shiraga, F. (2012). Enhanced depth imaging spectral-domain optical coherence tomography of subfoveal choroidal thickness in normal Japanese eyes. *Japan Journal of Ophthalmology*, 56(3), 230–235.

Margolis, R., & Spaide, R. F. (2009). A pilot study of enhanced depth imaging optical coherence tomography of the choroid in normal eyes. *American Journal of Ophthalmology*, 147(5), 811–815.

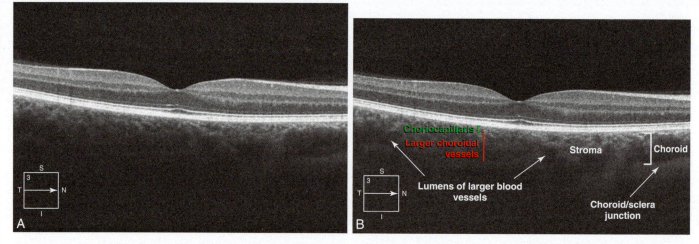

FIG. 3.1.1 Chorioretinal OCT images not using enhanced depth imaging (EDI) (A) and using EDI (B). (Courtesy of Carlos A. Moreira Neto.)

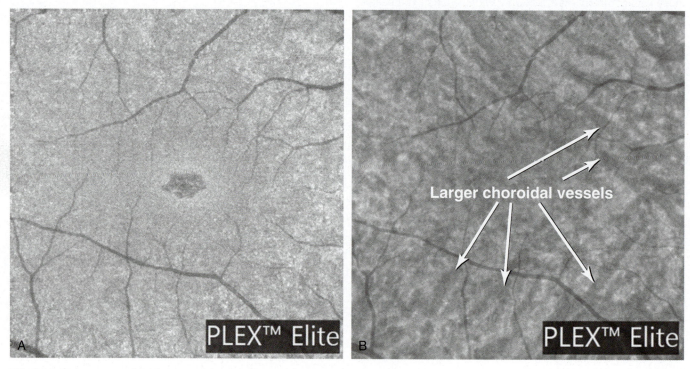

FIG. 3.1.2 En face structural OCT images of choriocapillaris (A) and Haller/Sattler layers (B).

Normal Vitreous
Nadia K. Waheed

4.1

Summary

Until recently, the anatomy of the vitreous could not be imaged in vivo. With the use of OCT, a better view and understanding of vitreous structure have become possible. Along with normal structure, abnormal vitreous processes such as vitreomacular traction have been revealed (Duker et al., 2013). High dynamic range imaging as well as enhanced vitreous imaging techniques present on most commercially available OCT devices allow visualization of the fluid-filled spaces as well as the collagenous and cellular structure of the vitreous. Secondary features of vitreous debris are also often identifiable on spectral domain (SD) OCT (Fig. 4.1.1).

Key OCT Features

In OCT of a normal retina, the following vitreous structures may be observed:

- Posterior cortical vitreous (posterior hyaloid) (Fig. 4.1.2)
- Retrohyaloid space: Created after posterior vitreous detachment (Fig. 4.1.2).
- Premacular bursa: Liquid space overlying the macula, caused by liquefaction of the vitreous (Fig. 4.1.3).

REFERENCE

Duker, J. S., Kaiser, P. K., Binder, S., de Smet, M. D., Gaudric, A., Reichel, E., et al. (2013). The International Vitreomacular Traction Study Group classification of vitreomacular adhesion, traction, and macular hole. *Ophthalmology*, *120*(12), 2611–2619.

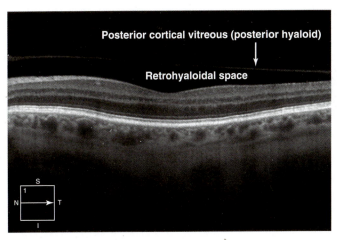

FIG. 4.1.2 Posterior hyaloid and retrohyaloid spaces.

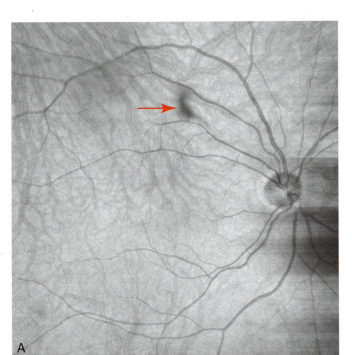

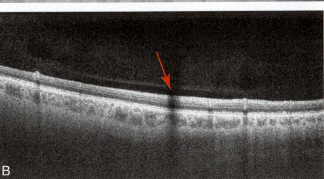

FIG. 4.1.1 Vitreous opacity *(arrows)* demonstrates shadowing on swept source OCT.

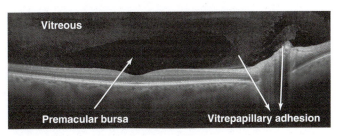

FIG. 4.1.3 Premacular bursa in a normal patient using spectral domain OCT.

OCT: Artifacts and Errors
Carlos A. Moreira Neto

5.1

Summary

Artifacts can occur during image acquisition or analysis because of patient, operator, or software factors. Accurate image interpretation depends on the quality of the image and an understanding of the various artifacts that can affect an OCT image (Duker et al., 2014).

Mirror Artifact

- Occurs only on spectral domain (SD) OCT.
- Occurs when the area of interest crosses the zero-delay line and results in an inverted image.
- Reasons:
  1. OCT device is pushed too close to the eye.
  2. Conditions in which the curvature of the retina is such that it crosses the zero-delay line, such as retinoschisis, retinal detachment, an elevated choroidal lesion, or high myopia (Fig. 5.1.1).

Vignetting

- Occurs when the iris blocks a part of the OCT beam.
- Loss of signal is seen over one side of the image (Fig. 5.1.2).

Misalignment

- This occurs when the fovea is not centered during the volumetric scan (Fig. 5.1.3).
- Most common reason is a patient with poor fixation or incorrect placement of fixation target by operator.

- The Early Treatment Diabetic Retinopathy Study (ETDRS) grid usually can be moved to get an accurate measure of the foveal thickness

Software Breakdown

- OCT segmentation lines are incorrectly drawn because there is misidentification of the inner or outer retinal boundaries.
- Vitreomacular surface disorders (epiretinal membrane, vitreomacular traction) could cause inner line breakdown.
- Outer retinal/retinal pigment epithelium disorders (age macular degeneration, cystoid macular edema) might cause outer line breakdown (Fig. 5.1.4).

Blink Artifact

- If a patient blinks during image acquisition, loss of data occurs.
- OCT scans and volumetric maps both show black or white horizontal bars (Fig. 5.1.5).

Motion Artifact

- Occurs when there is movement of the eye during the scan acquisition.
- OCT image shows distortion or double scanning of the same area.
- Blood vessels are misaligned (Fig. 5.1.6).
- The fovea may be duplicated.
- This is much less common due to better eye tracking software on current machines.

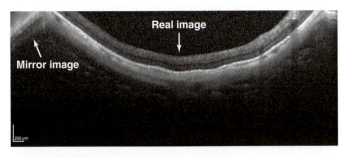

FIG. 5.1.1 Mirror artifact occurring in a high myopic eye.

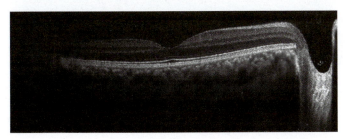

FIG. 5.1.2 Vignetting: loss of signal over the left side of the image.

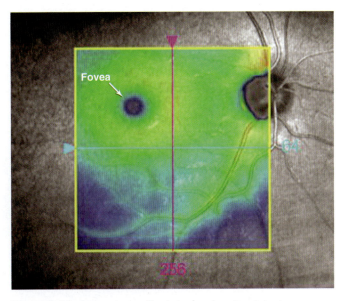

FIG. 5.1.3 Misalignment error. The fovea is not centered due to an eccentric fixation.

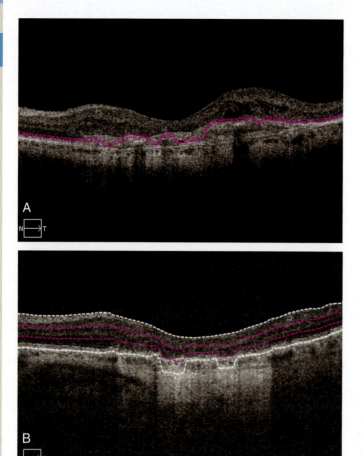

FIG. 5.1.4 Software breakdown caused by choroidal neovascularization (A) and geographic atrophy (B).

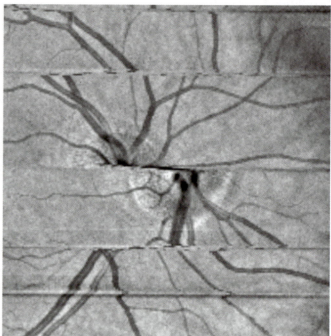

FIG. 5.1.6 Motion artifact.

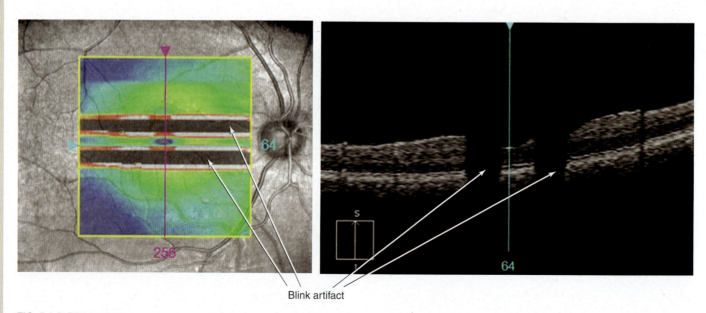

Blink artifact

FIG. 5.1.5 Blink artifact.

Out-of-Range Error

- Occurs when the B-scan is not centered in the preview screen, resulting in it being shifted out of the scanning range
- A section of the OCT scan is cut off (Fig. 5.1.7).

REFERENCE

Duker, J. S., Waheed, N. K., & Goldman, D. R. (2014). Artifacts on OCT. *Handbook of retinal OCT*. St. Louis: Elsevier; 2014.

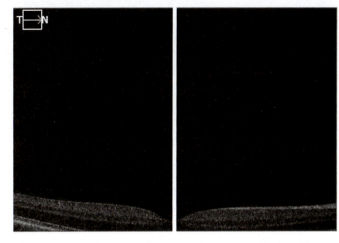

FIG. 5.1.7 Out-of-range error. Because of improper positioning of the machine during image acquisition, the outer retina and the choroid image is cut off.

Artifacts are very common in OCT angiography and their identification is important for appropriate image interpretation (Ferrara et al., 2016).

Blockage Artifacts (Fig. 5.2.1)

- Blockage artifacts are caused by lesions that affect light penetration through ocular tissues, including both the anterior and posterior segments.
- Anterior segment blockage can be cause by cataract, inflammation, or corneal scar.
- Posterior segment blockage can be caused by intravitreal hemorrhage or inflammation, floaters, intraretinal or subretinal hemorrhage, pigment epithelial detachment (PED), or large drusen.

White Line Artifacts (Fig. 5.2.2)

- Caused by transverse ocular movements.
- A major cause of artifacts in OCT angiography.

False Positive Flow

- Ocular movements are in the axial direction (arterial pulsation).
- An OCT dataset may be displaced and may have enough decorrelation to cause the appearance of flow (Ferrara et al., 2016; Spaide et al., 2015).

Quilting Defect (Fig. 5.2.3)

- Related to software correction of ocular movement.
- Caused by multiple saccades in the horizontal and vertical directions.

False Negative Flow

- Caused by blood flow below a given threshold.
- Vessels seem absent even if they are present.

Projection Artifact (Fig. 5.2.4)

- Superficial vessels are seen in deep and choroidal slabs when they are not actually present in those slabs (Ferrara et al., 2016; Spaide et al., 2015).

Vessel Suplication (Fig. 5.2.5)

- Result of a breakdown in registration of the X and Y scans.
- Caused by eye movement.

Segmentation Errors (Fig. 5.2.6)

- Caused by PED, macular edema, or other pathologic process that disrupts the horizontal alignment of retinal layers.

Shadowing Artifact (Fig. 5.2.7)

- Usually appears in the choriocapillary segmentation.
- Caused by PED, hemorrhage, floaters.

Wide-Field Artifacts (Fig. 5.2.8)

- Represented by artifacts that appear only in wide-field OCT angiography (OCTA) images (12 × 12–18 × 18) (such as alignment errors and eyelash artifacts) and higher prevalence of general alterations (such as motion artifacts, segmentation errors, and defocus).
- Can be related to anatomic-functional alterations of peripheral retina due to retinal curvature or differences in axial length.

REFERENCES

Ferrara, D., Waheed, N. K., & Duker, J. S. (2016). Investigating the choriocapillaris and choroidal vasculature with new optical coherence tomography technologies. *Progress in Retinal Eye Research*, *52*, 130–155.

Spaide, R. F., Fujimoto, J. G., & Waheed, N. K. (2015). Image artifacts in optical coherence tomography angiography. *Retina*, *35*(11), 2163–2180.

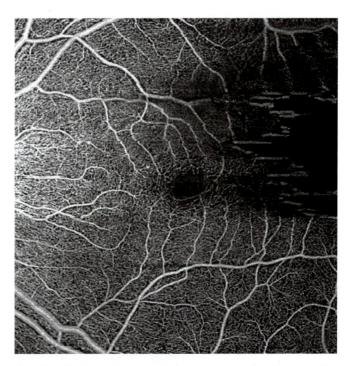

FIG. 5.2.1 Blockage artifact causing a focal loss of signal. (Courtesy of Carlos A. Moreira Neto.)

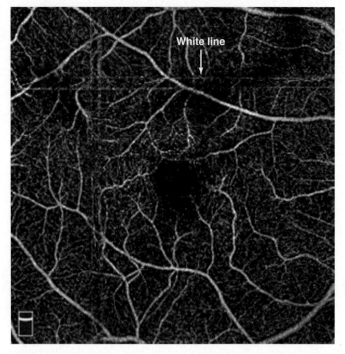

FIG. 5.2.2 White line artifact. (Courtesy of Carlos A. Moreira Neto.)

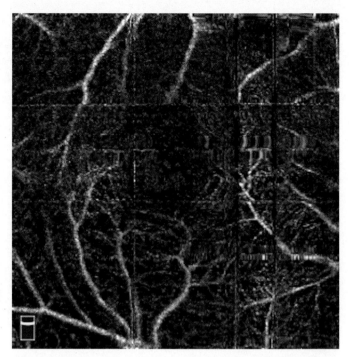

FIG. 5.2.3 Quilting artifact.

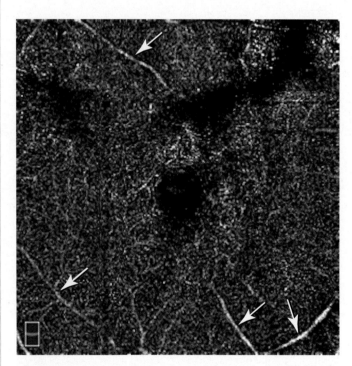

FIG. 5.2.4 Projection artifact on deep plexus. Vessels from the superficial plexus *(arrows)* are seen in the deep plexus. (Courtesy of Carlos A. Moreira Neto.)

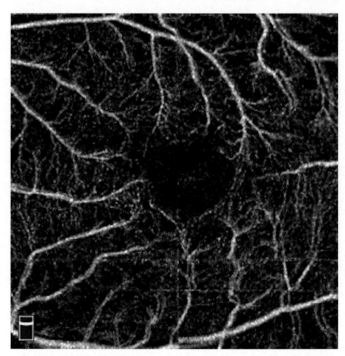

FIG. 5.2.5 Vessel duplication.

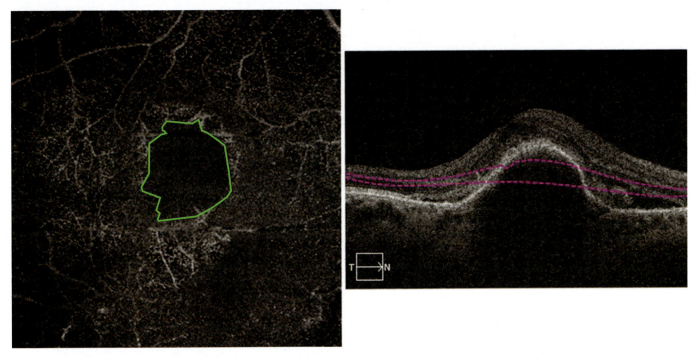

FIG. 5.2.6 Segmentation error *(green line)* caused by a pigment epithelial detachment.

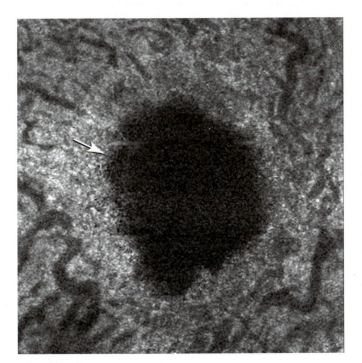

FIG. 5.2.7 Shadowing artifact *(arrows)* in the choriocapillaris segmentation.

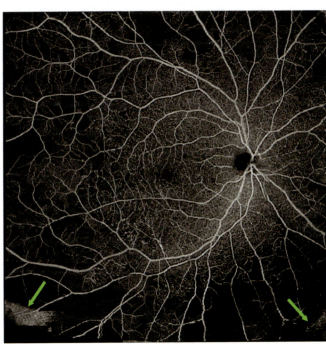

FIG. 5.2.8 Anatomic-functional characteristics causing errors of the peripheral retina due to retinal curvature *(arrows)*.

Drusen
Ivana N. Despotovic

6.1.1

Summary

Drusen are focal extracellular lipid-rich deposits located between the basal lamina of retinal pigment epithelium (RPE) and the inner collagenous layer of Bruch's membrane (BM) (Curcio, 2018). Drusen may range in appearance, size, and location, and they are distinguishable by multimodal imaging. By OCT, hard drusen and cuticular drusen have steep sides (Fig. 6.1.1.1), while soft drusen are dome shaped with sloping sides (Figs. 6.1.1.2 and 6.1.1.3). Soft drusen have homogenous and "ground-glass" moderate internal reflectivity. (Fig. 6.1.1.2) (Curcio, 2018). Cuticular drusen have a spheroid or triangular shape, with RPE attenuation at the apices, and they present as a saw-tooth pattern on OCT (Fig. 6.1.1.1) (Balaratnasingam et al., 2018).

Drusen can enlarge, followed by anterior RPE migration (Fig. 6.1.1.3) on top of drusen (hyperreflective foci on OCT), collapse, and atrophy (Curcio, 2018). Approximately 10% of soft drusen may have subclinical (nonexudative) neovascularization on OCT angiography (OCTA) (Roisman et al., 2016). The presence of nonexudative macular neovascularization (MNV) in intermediate age-related macular degeneration (AMD) is a risk factor for progression to exudative AMD (de Oliveira Dias et al., 2018). On the other hand, drusen or drusenoid pigment epithelial detachment (PED) can be accompanied by subretinal fluid (SRF) in the absence of MNV and may be the result of RPE decompensation (Hilely et al., 2021).

OCT imaging of refractile drusen (drusenoid material containing small refractile spherules) (Fig. 6.1.1.4) shows hyperreflective dots (many small spherules rich in calcium phosphate) and appear to be a stage of drusen regression marked by loss of RPE, thus contributing to the development of geographic atrophy (GA) (Suzuki et al., 2015).

Subretinal drusenoid deposits (SDDs), also known as reticular pseudodrusen (Figs. 6.1.1.3 and 6.1.1.5) can be confounded with drusen, but are actually a clinically distinct entity located above the RPE (between RPE and photoreceptors).

The tomographic features of drusen on OCT have been extensively investigated in natural history studies as potential biomarkers for AMD progression, although some features have yet to be validated. Drusen size and confluency have been historically associated with the progression of AMD. More recently, OCTA has become a useful imaging tool for identifying and monitoring subclinical MNV in nonexudative AMD. OCTA analysis of choriocapillaris perfusion in patients with nonexudative AMD is currently limited to the research setting, but may be used in clinical practice in the future (Fig. 6.1.1.3).

Key Points

- A few small hard drusen are considered normal aging and do not represent a risk for progression to advanced AMD.
- The presence of large, soft drusen represents a high probability for the development of GA and choroidal neovascularization.
- Hyperreflective foci (pigment migration) are correlated with an increased risk of progression to GA.
- SDDs (also known as reticular pseudodrusen) are located above the RPE and are associated with progression to advanced AMD.

REFERENCES

Balaratnasingam, C., Cherepanoff, S., Dolz-Marco, R., Killingsworth, M., Chen, F. K., Mendis, R., et al. (2018). Cuticular drusen: Clinical phenotypes and natural course defined using multimodal imaging. *Ophthalmology*, *125*, 100–118.

Curcio, C. A. (2018). Soft drusen in age-related macular degeneration: Biology and targeting via the oil spill strategies. *Investigative Ophthalmology & Visual Science*, *59*(4), 160–181.

de Oliveira Dias, J. R., Zhang, Q., Garcia, J. M. B., Zheng, F., Motulsky, E. F., Roisman, L., et al. (2018). Natural history of subclinical neovascularization in nonexudative age-related macular degeneration using swept-source OCT angiography. *Ophthalmology*, *125*(2), 255–266.

Hilely, A., Au, A., Freund, K. B., Loewenstein, A., Souied, E. H., Zur, D., et al. (2021). Non-neovascular age-related macular degeneration with subretinal fluid. *British Journal of Ophthalmology*, *105*(10), 1415–1420. https://doi.org/10.1136/bjophthalmol-2020-317326. PMID: 32920528.

Roisman, L., Zhang, Q., Wang, R. K., Gregori, G., Zhang, A., Chen, C. -L., et al. (2016). Optical coherence tomography angiography of asymptomatic neovascularization in intermediate age-related macular degeneration. *Ophthalmology*, *123*, 1309–1319.

Suzuki, M., Curcio, C. A., Mullins, R. F., & Spaide, R. F. (2015). Refractile drusen: Clinical imaging and candidate histology. *Retina*, *35*(5), 859–865. https://doi.org/10.1097/IAE.0000000000000503.

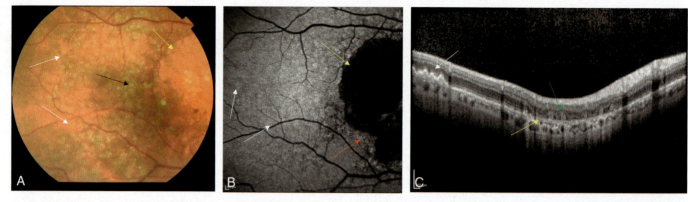

FIG. 6.1.1.1 Multimodal imaging of cuticular drusen in a patient with geographic atrophy (GA). (A) Color fundus photograph reveals the cuticular drusen as clusters of pale and yellow punctate lesions *(white arrows)* that coalesces into larger soft drusen on the right *(black arrow)*. GA involving the fovea is visible as a sharply demarcated depigmentation of the retinal pigment epithelium (RPE) with visible underlying choroidal vessels *(yellow arrow)*. (B) Fundus autofluorescence demonstrates a hypoautofluorescent center with a surrounding rim of hyperautofluorescence *(white arrows)*. The GA is visible as a hypoautofluorescence in the atrophic area *(yellow arrow)*, with a hyperautofluorescence around the GA borders *(red arrow)*. (C) OCT B-scan shows closely packed triangular sub-RPE elevations *(white arrow)* and GA *(yellow arrow)* associated with outer retinal tubulations (ORTs) *(green arrow)*. GA lesion is visualized as a loss of outer retinal layers and RPE, with underlying choroidal hypertransmission. ORTs are identified as hyperreflective circular structures with a hyporeflective center, located in the outer nuclear layer.

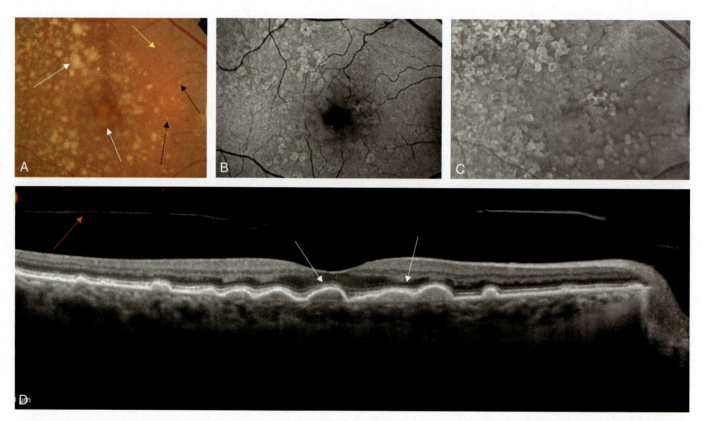

FIG. 6.1.1.2 Multimodal imaging of the soft drusen. (A) Color fundus photograph with the multiple, confluent, large, soft drusen *(white arrows)*. Small hard drusen are present, as well *(black arrows)*. Epiretinal membrane is barely visible superior-nasal to the macula *(yellow arrow)*. (B) Fundus autofluorescence and (C) near infrared image of the same eye. (D) OCT B-scan shows the confluent, large, soft drusen *(white arrows)*. A posterior hyaloid membrane is also visible *(red arrow)*.

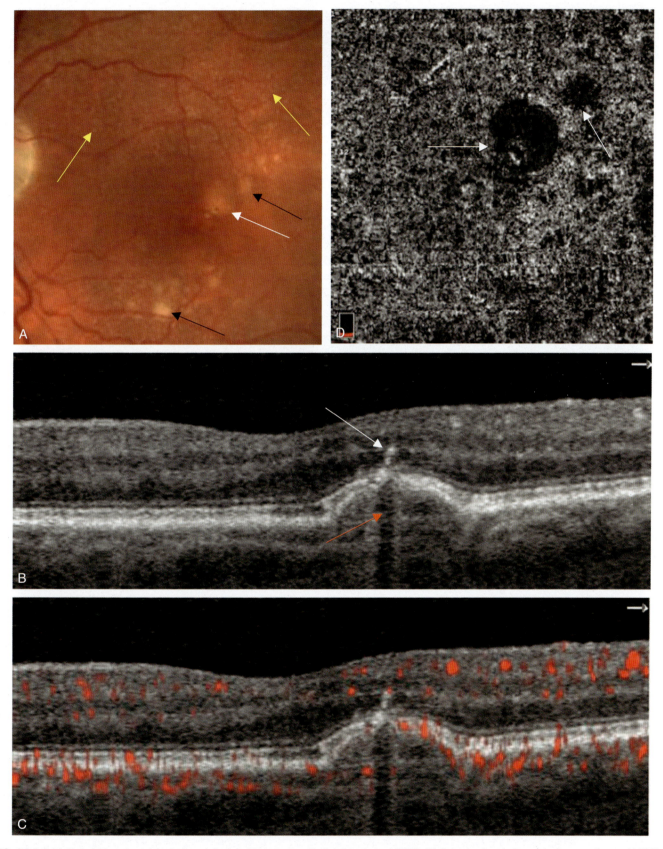

FIG. 6.1.1.3 Multimodal imaging of a parafoveal drusenoid pigment epithelial detachment (PED). (A) Color fundus photograph shows a drusenoid PED with hyperpigmentation *(white arrow)*, multiple large soft drusen with indistinct margins *(black arrows)* and subretinal drusenoid deposits *(yellow arrows)*. (B) Cross-sectional OCT scan demonstrates a drusenoid PED with homogenous, moderate internal reflectivity and hyperreflective foci *(white arrow)* on the top of PED. The hyperreflective foci are associated with a shadowing beneath *(red arrow)*. (C) OCTA B-scan with flow overlay does not show a flow signal within the PED, implying an absence of macular neovascularization. (D) OCTA 3 × 3 mm at the choriocapillaris (CC) level demonstrates the areas of decreased signal in the choriocapillaris (due to a shadowing artifact) underlying the PED and drusen *(white arrows)*. It is difficult to assess the presence of flow impairment. No neovascular network is noted.

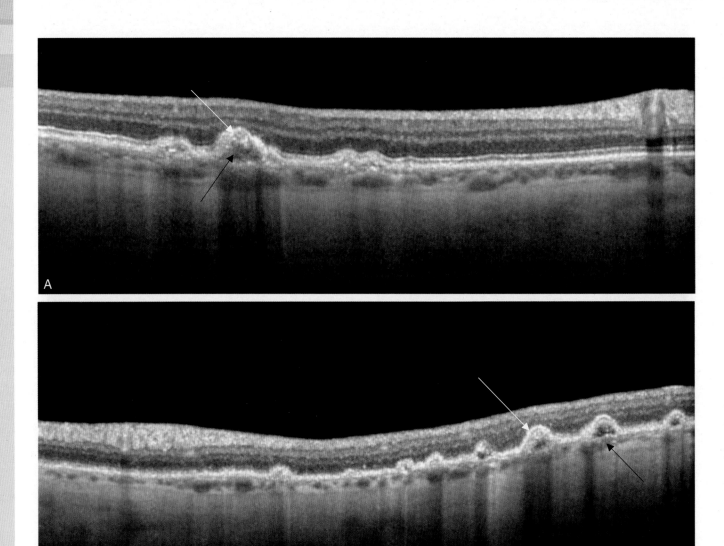

FIG. 6.1.1.4 OCT B-scans of refractile drusen, containing small refractile spherules-hyperreflective dots *(white arrows)* and hyporeflective cores *(black arrows)*.

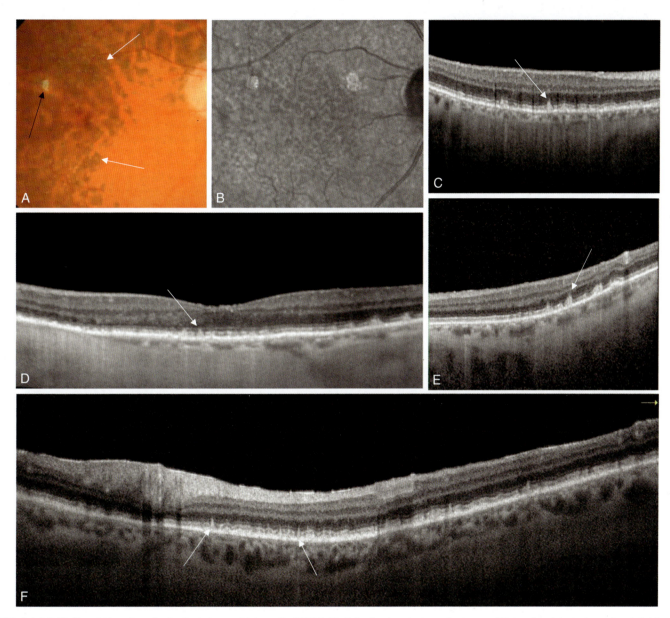

FIG. 6.1.1.5 Multimodal imaging of subretinal drusenoid deposits (SDDs). (A) Color fundus photograph shows whitish-yellow interlacing network *(white arrow)*. A refractile druse is visible on the left *(black arrow)*. (B) On near infrared image, the lesions appear isoreflectant and are surrounded by halos of hyporeflectance. (C, D, E, and F) Cross-sectional OCT scans of the different eyes identify late-stage SDD as well-defined triangular hyperreflective deposits breaking through the ellipsoid zone *(white arrows)*.

Geographic Atrophy

6.1.2

Ivana N. Despotovic

Summary

Geographic atrophy (GA) is a manifestation of late-stage non-neovascular age-related macular degeneration (AMD). By OCT, the GA lesion is visualized as a loss of outer retinal layers and retinal pigment epithelium (RPE), with underlying choroidal hypertransmission, resulting from a loss of absorbing structures (Figs. 6.1.2.1–6.1.2.3). Loss of the outer retina causes subsidence of the inner nuclear layer (INL) and outer plexiform layer (OPL). The wedge-shaped hyporeflectivity between the Bruch membrane and the outer plexiform layer may become visible (Querques et al., 2015). Outer retinal tubulation (ORT) is a display of photoreceptor rearrangement after retinal injury and is commonly found in advanced AMD. It may be identified on cross-sectional OCT scans as a hyperreflective circular or ovoid structure with a hyporeflective center (Fig. 6.1.2.2), located in the outer nuclear layer (Zweifel et al., 2009).

The early signs of atrophy, which are not clinically detectable, can be visualized on the OCT. In complete RPE and outer retinal atrophy (cRORA), there must be a loss of outer retinal layers, RPE loss, and choroidal hypertransmission of at least 250 μm. In incomplete RPE and outer retinal atrophy (iRORA) (Figs. 6.1.2.4 and 6.1.2.5), these OCT signs are present but do not fulfill all the size criteria for cRORA (Guymer et al., 2020).

Natural history studies have strived to identify predictive biomarkers of AMD progression. Large soft drusen (Figs. 6.1.2.1 and 6.1.2.5) are associated with a high risk for progression to GA (Ferris et al., 2005). Intraretinal hyperreflective foci (Christenbury et al., 2013), heterogeneous internal reflectivity of drusen (Fig. 6.1.2.4) (Veerappan et al., 2016), and subretinal drusenoid deposits (SDDs) (Zweifel et al., 2010) are among the OCT biomarkers of atrophy development. Drusen regression (Figs. 6.1.2.4 and 6.1.2.5) may be a sign of progression toward GA (Schlanitz et al., 2017).

OCT angiography (OCTA) is a rapid and noninvasive method for identifying and monitoring subclinical macular neovascularization (MNV) in eyes with nonexudative AMD. In the research setting, this imaging modality is used in a choriocapillaris (CC) flow deficit assessment in GA patients (Fig. 6.1.2.6) (Waheed et al., 2016).

Key Points

- GA is characterized on OCT by atrophy of the outer nuclear layer, external limiting membrane (ELM), ellipsoid zone (EZ), photoreceptors, RPE, and CC, accompanied by choroidal hypertransmission.

- iRORA is a recently described entity, based on the specific OCT features, that predicts the development of cRORA (GA correlate).
- Large soft drusen, intraretinal hyperreflective foci, drusen regression, and SDDs are some of the OCT biomarkers of GA development.
- A subclinical MNV in eyes with nonexudative AMD may be identified and monitored by the OCTA.

REFERENCES

Christenbury, J. G., Folgar, F. A., O'Connell, R. V., Chiu, S. J., Farsiu, S., Toth, C. A., et al. (2013). Progression of intermediate age-related macular degeneration with proliferation and inner retinal migration of hyperreflective foci. *Ophthalmology, 120*, 1038–1045.

Ferris, F. L., Davis, M. D., Clemons, T. E., Lee, L. -Y., Chew, E. Y., Lindblad, A. S., et al. (2005). A simplified severity scale for age-related macular degeneration: AREDS Report No. 18. *Archives of Ophthalmology, 123*, 1570–1574.

Guymer, R. H., Rosenfeld, P. J., Curcio, C. A., Holz, F. G., Staurenghi, G., Freund, K. B., et al. (2020). Incomplete retinal pigment epithelial and outer retinal atrophy in age-related macular degeneration: Classification of Atrophy Meeting report 4. *Ophthalmology, 127*, 394–409.

Querques, G., Capuano, V., Frascio, P., Zweifel, S., Georges, A., & Souied, E. H. (2015). Wedge-shaped subretinal hyporeflectivity in geographic atrophy. *Retina, 35*, 1735–1742.

Schlanitz, F. G., Baumann, B., Kundi, M., Sacu, S., Baratsits, M., Scheschy, U., et al. (2017). Drusen volume development over time and its relevance to the course of age-related macular degeneration. *British Journal of Ophthalmology, 101*(2), 198–203. https://doi.org/10.1136/bjophthalmol-2016-308422. pii: bjophthalmol-2016-308422.

Veerappan, M., El-Hage-Sleiman, A. -K. M., Tai, V., Chiu, S. J., Winter, K. P., Stinnett, S. S., et al. (2016). Optical coherence tomography reflective drusen substructures predict progression to geographic atrophy in age-related macular degeneration. *Ophthalmology, 123*, 2554–2570.

Waheed, N. K., Moult, E. M., Fujimoto, J. G., & Rosenfeld, P. J. (2016). Optical coherence tomography angiography of dry age-related macular degeneration. *Developments in Ophthalmology, 56*, 91–100.

Zweifel, S. A., Engelbert, M., Laud, K., Margolis, R., Spaide, R. F., & Freund, K. B. (2009). Outer retinal tubulation: A novel optical coherence tomography finding. *Archives of Ophthalmology, 127*(12), 1596–1602. https://doi.org/10.1001/archophthalmol.2009.326.

Zweifel, S. A., Imamura, Y., Spaide, T. C., Fujiwara, T., & Spaide, R. F. (2010). Prevalence and significance of subretinal drusenoid deposits (reticular pseudodrusen) in age-related macular degeneration. *Ophthalmology, 117*, 1775–1781.

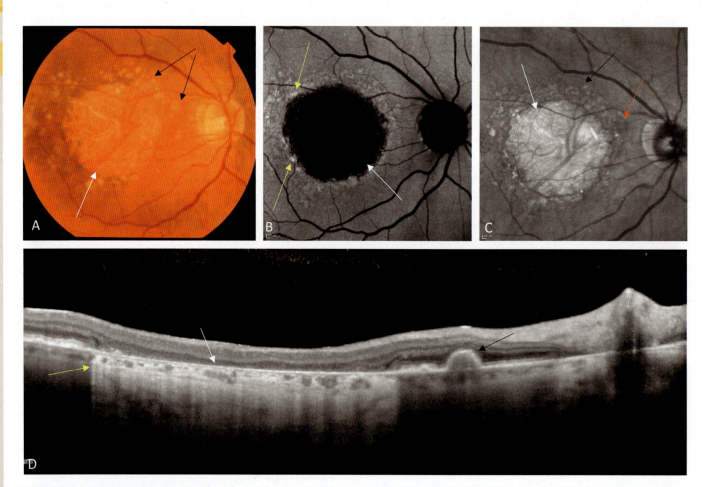

FIG. 6.1.2.1 A multimodal imaging of unifocal geographic atrophy (GA), involving the fovea. (A) Color fundus photograph of a GA secondary to age-related macular degeneration involving the center of the fovea, with a sharply demarcated area of retinal pigment epithelium (RPE) depigmentation with visible choroidal vessels *(white arrow)*. It is surrounded by large, confluent, soft drusen *(black arrows)*. (B) Fundus autofluorescence demonstrates a hypoautofluorescence in the atrophic area *(white arrow)*, with a hyperautofluorescence around the GA borders *(yellow arrows)*. (C) Near-infrared image reveals a well-demarcated, bright zone of hyperreflectance *(white arrow)*. The hyperreflective drusen are visible *(black arrow)*. The large druse depicted on the OCT B-scan is hyporeflective *(red arrow)*. (D) A cross-sectional OCT scan shows the loss of RPE in the area of GA, with a depression of the inner retinal layers as the outer retinal layers are lost, and increased visibility of Bruch's membrane and the choroid *(white arrow)*. The OCT signal is increased below the level of RPE, corresponding to a hypertransmission effect *(yellow arrow)*. The large soft druse is visible on the right *(black arrow)*.

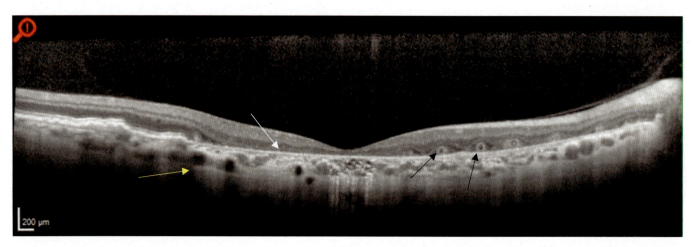

FIG. 6.1.2.2 A cross-sectional OCT scan shows the loss of outer nuclear layer, photoreceptors, and retinal pigment epithelium in the area of geographic atrophy, with thinning of the neurosensory retina *(white arrow)*. The hypertransmission effect is present *(yellow arrow)*. On the right side of the scan, the ORTs are visible *(black arrows)*.

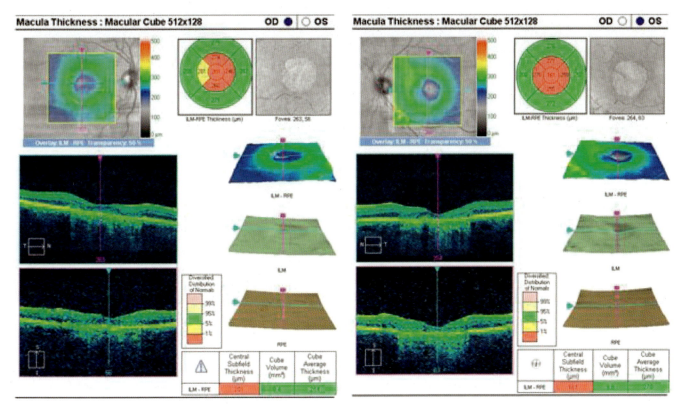

FIG. 6.1.2.3 Macular cube scan showing thickness maps, en face OCT, and cross-sectional OCT scans. Decreased thickness is evident in the center of the macula. En face OCT shows the area of geographic atrophy (GA). Cross-sectional OCT scan demonstrates a loss of the outer retinal layers and retinal pigment epithelium (*RPE*) in the areas of GA, causing thinning of the neurosensory retina. The OCT signal is increased below the level of the RPE, corresponding to the hypertransmission effect. *ILM*, Internal limiting membrane; *OD*, oculus dexter (right eye); *OS*, oculus sinister (left eye).

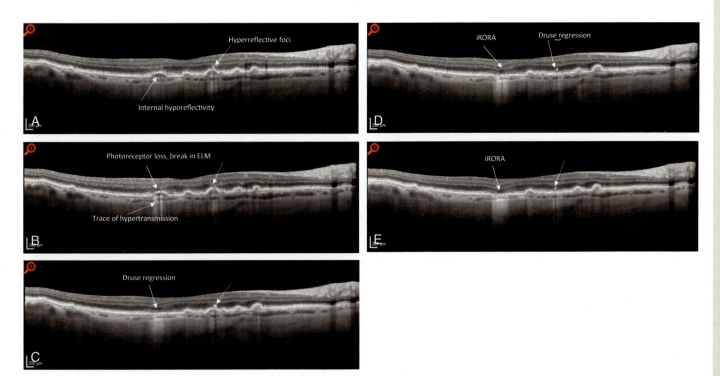

FIG. 6.1.2.4 Cross-sectional OCT scans demonstrate drusen regression and progression to the iRORA over the course of 14 months. (A) Soft drusen are present, with the far left druse, showing an internal hyporeflectivity. (B) Loss of the photoreceptors and break in the external limiting membrane (ELM), above the same druse, and the traces of an increased transmission below. (C) Druse regression occurs. (D) OCT scan reveals iRORA, measuring 101 μm, and (E) progresses to 180 μm diameter, still falling under the iRORA definition. *iRORA*, Incomplete retinal pigment epithelium and outer retinal atrophy.

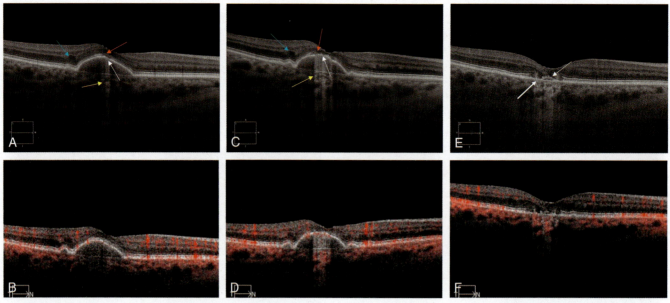

FIG. 6.1.2.5 The horizontal B-scans (A, C, and E) and OCTA B-scans (B, D, and F) demonstrate a regression of the large drusenoid subfoveal pigment epithelial detachment (PED), progressing to the atrophy, over a 1-year period. A subfoveal dome-shaped elevation of the hyperreflective retinal pigment epithelium (RPE) layer over a homogenous moderate internal reflective space, showing some loss of the RPE and photoreceptors *(white arrow)*, with a trace of a hypertransmission signal *(yellow arrow)*. The external limiting membrane (ELM) is preserved *(red arrow)*. A small cystoid space is present on the left *(blue arrow)* (A). The loss of the RPE and photoreceptors progresses *(white arrow)*, with a visible choroidal hypertransmission *(yellow arrow)*. The ELM is disrupted *(red arrow)*. The cystoid space is still visible *(blue arrow)* (C). The PED collapses, leading to incomplete retinal pigment epithelium and outer retinal atrophy development (<250 μm, *thick white arrow*). Some RPE is still preserved (E). OCTA B-scans with flow overlay (B, D, and F) do not show a flow signal within the PED, implying an absence of macular neovascularization.

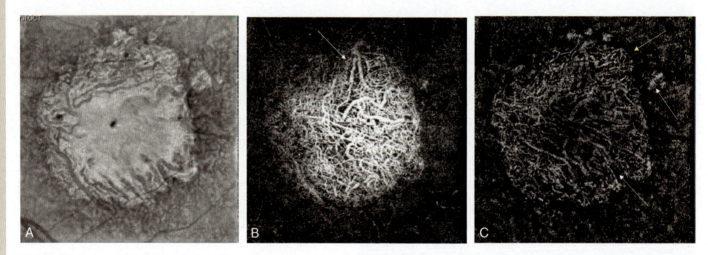

FIG. 6.1.2.6 En face OCTA 6 × 6 mm of a multifocal geographic atrophy (GA) with a foveal involvement. No evidence of macular neovascularization. (A) Choriocapillaris (CC) structural OCT reveals a GA lesion. (B) Avascular and (C) CC slabs allow visualization of the larger choroidal vessels that rest below the GA *(white arrows)*. CC slab demonstrates a CC impairment around the GA border *(yellow arrow)*.

Isolated Pigment Epithelial Detachment

Ivana N. Despotovic

6.1.3

Summary

Retinal pigment epithelial detachment (PED) results from a separation between the retinal pigment epithelium (RPE) basement membrane and the inner collagenous layer of Bruch's membrane. Although often associated with an underlying disorder, PED may occasionally be an isolated finding (Figs. 6.1.3.1 and 6.1.3.2) with no known primary diagnosis. Idiopathic PEDs tend to be multifocal, small, and bilateral (Gass et al., 2005). An isolated PED may be clinically insignificant, or it may represent an intermediate stage between pachychoroid (Figs. 6.1.3.1A,B and 6.1.3.2B–D) and classic central serous chorioretinopathy (CSC) (Arif et al., 2018).

OCT features of an isolated PED usually include a well-demarcated, abrupt, dome-shaped elevation of the hyperreflective RPE layer lining over an optically clear or homogenous-hyporeflective space (Figs. 6.1.3.1B and 6.1.3.2B–D). It can resolve completely, sometimes leaving RPE atrophy.

An isolated PED needs to be observed because of a risk of choroidal neovascularization (CNV). A heterogeneous-hyperreflective material under the RPE may represent vascularized PED. The use of OCT angiography (OCTA) in association with OCT (Figs. 6.1.3.1 B, 6.1.3.2B–D, and 6.1.3.3) scans may lead to early detection of shallow type 1 CNV in an isolated PED.

Key Points

- Isolated PED is not associated with a known underlying condition and is usually asymptomatic.
- It may be clinically irrelevant, or suggest intermediate stage between pachychoroid and classic CSC, and should be followed closely because of the potential risk for development of CNV. OCTA is a useful tool in the screening for CNV in an isolated PED.

REFERENCES

Arif, F., Pryds, A., & Larsen, M. (2018). Isolated pigment epithelium detachment: evidence for relation to central serous chorioretinopathy and effect of photodynamic therapy. *Acta Ophthalmologica*, *96*(8), 821–827. https://doi.org/10.1111/aos.13838.

Gass, J. D., Bressler, S. B., Akduman, L., Olk, J., Caskey, P. J., & Zimmerman, L. E. (2005). Bilateral idiopathic multifocal retinal pigment epithelium detachments in otherwise healthy middle-aged adults: a clinicopathologic study. *Retina*, *25*, 304–310.

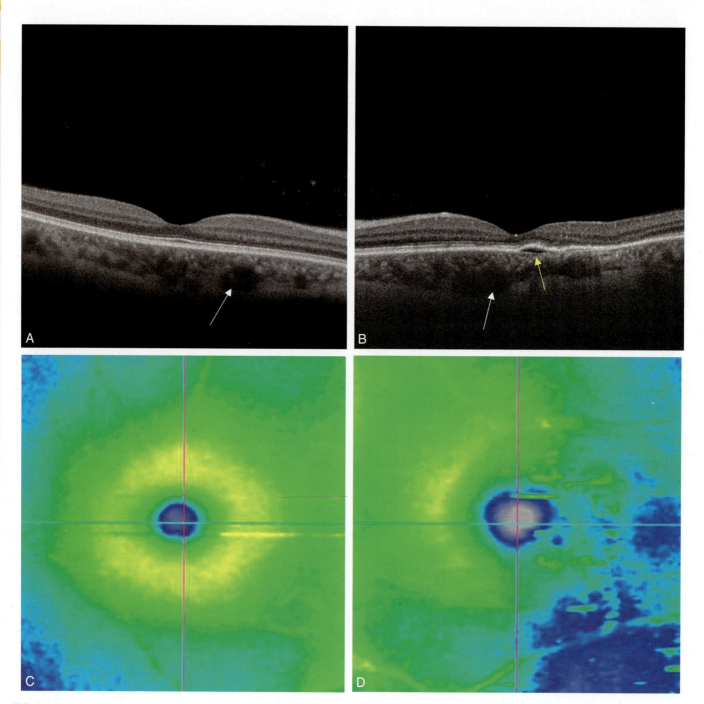

FIG. 6.1.3.1 An isolated pigment epithelial detachment (PED) in an asymptomatic 43-year-old male patient. Cross-sectional OCT shows the thick choroid (subfoveal choroidal thickness measured 381 μm in the right eye) and pachyvessels *(white arrows)* in both eyes (A) and (B). The left eye demonstrates a small, subfoveal, low-lying PED, with a normal foveal contour *(yellow arrow)*. No intraretinal fluid or subretinal fluid present (B). Normal thickness map in the right eye (C) and slight decrease of foveal thickness (due to a PED impact) and inferior temporal thickness in the left eye (D).

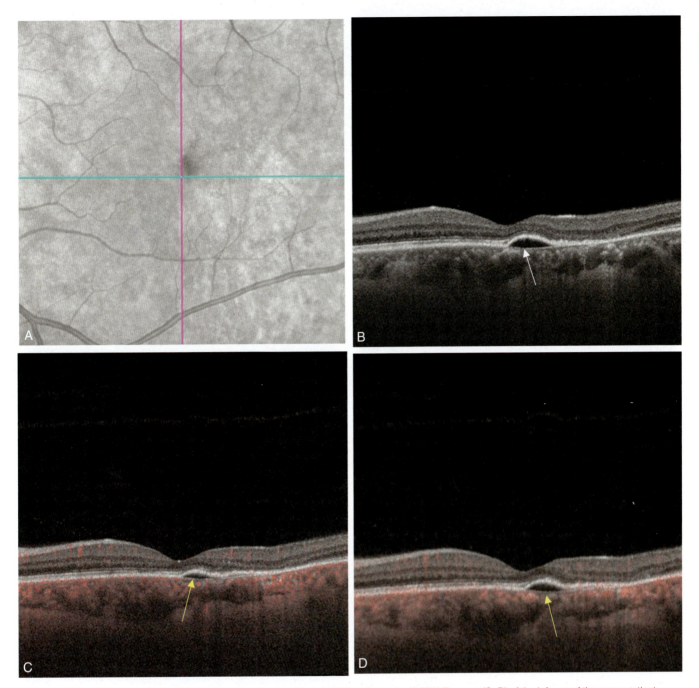

FIG. 6.1.3.2 Structural OCT en face (A) and horizontal B-scan (B) and OCT angiography (OCTA) B-scans (C, D) of the left eye of the same patient depicted in Fig. 6.1.3.1. B-scans reveal a subfoveal elevation of the hyperreflective retinal pigment epithelium (RPE) layer over a homogenous-hyporeflective space *(white arrow)*. RPE is intact. Thick choroid is present. OCTA B-scans with flow overlay do not show a flow signal within the PED *(yellow arrow)*, implying an absence of choroidal neovascularization (C and D).

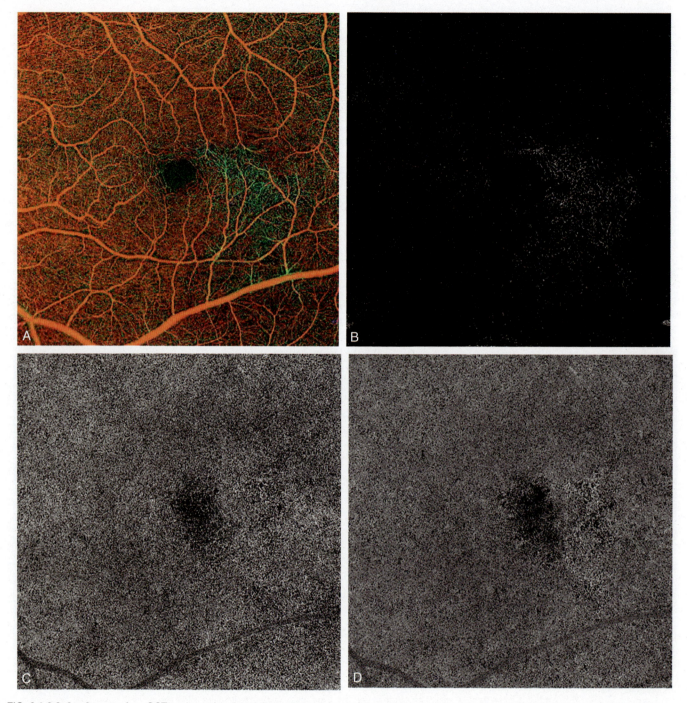

FIG. 6.1.3.3 6 × 6 mm en face OCT angiography of the left eye of the same patient as in Figs. 6.1.3.1 and 6.1.3.2. Retina depth encoded slab (A). Avascular (B), ORCC (C), and choriocapillaris (CC) slabs do not show evidence of a choroidal neovascularization (D). *ORRC*, Outer retina to CC.

Type 1 Macular Neovascular Membrane

A. Yasin Alibhai*

6.2.1

Summary

Type 1 macular neovascularization (MNV) involves the formation of abnormal blood vessels that develop from the choroid, extend through the Bruch's membrane, and arborize beneath the retinal pigment epithelium (RPE). On fluorescein angiography, type 1 MNV is characterized as "occult choroidal neovascularization (CNV)," manifesting as stippled fluorescence (leakage from undetermined source) or as fibrovascular pigment epithelial detachment (PED) (Fig. 6.2.1.1).

These neovascular lesions are commonly associated with age-related macular degeneration (AMD). They can, however, also develop because of other pathologic processes, such as central serous chorioretinopathy (CSC).

Type 1 MNV lies within the sub-RPE space and results in elevation of the overlying RPE. The most characteristic OCT findings include irregular PEDs, occasionally with thickening of the overlying RPE (Figs. 6.2.1.2 and 6.2.1.3). These PEDs may present with variable internal reflectivity, ranging from hyporeflective or optically empty spaces to hyperreflective, usually heterogeneous internal reflectivity. On OCT scans with high quality, the intravascular lumens of the MNV complex may be documented, giving the appearance of "stacked" material. In active, exudative MNVs, associated subretinal and/or intraretinal fluid may also be present (Keane et al., 2012).

The diagnosis of inactive, nonexudative type 1 MNVs may be challenging because they can be confounded with drusenoid PED or nonneovascular PED (Fig. 6.2.1.4). On OCT, they commonly appear as small PEDs with increased internal reflectivity. The nonexudative neovascular complex can be identified only with OCT angiography (OCTA) (Roisman et al., 2016).

On OCTA imaging, type 1 MNVs can often be visualized within the PED as abnormal vessels that lie between the RPE and Bruch's membrane. The neovascular complex can have many different appearances but typically consists of thicker central vessels and finer peripheral vessels (Fig. 6.2.1.5). Associated choriocapillaris loss can usually be seen in the surrounding regions on OCTA (Spaide et al., 2018). Long-term follow-up with OCTA has shown that the majority of type 1 MNV lesions continue to grow despite ongoing treatment with anti-vascular endothelial growth factor agents (Xu et al., 2018).

Key Points

- Type 1 MNV is classified based on its anatomic location, being present above Bruch's membrane but below the RPE.
- On OCT, type 1 MNV manifests as PED and commonly multilobulated with variable internal reflectivity.
- On fluorescein angiography, type 1 MNV manifests as "occult CNV," with stippled fluorescence or fibrovascular PED.
- On OCT angiography, type 1 MNV appears as a network of vessels lying between the RPE and Bruch's membrane.
- Type 1 MNV is commonly associated with AMD, but they can also be secondary to other conditions such as trauma, CSC, and pseudoxanthoma elasticum.

REFERENCES

Keane, P. A., Patel, P. J., Liakopoulos, S., Heussen, F. M., Sadda, S. R., & Tufail, A. (2012). Evaluation of age-related macular degeneration with optical coherence tomography. *Surv Ophthalmol*, 57, 389–414.

Roisman, L., Zhang, Q., Wang, R. K., Gregori, G., Zhang, A., Chen, C. -L., et al. (2016). Optical coherence tomography angiography of asymptomatic neovascularization in intermediate age-related macular degeneration. *Ophthalmology*, 123(6), 1309–1319. https://doi.org/10.1016/j.ophtha.2016.01.044.

Spaide, R. F., Fujimoto, J. G., Waheed, N. K., Sadda, S. R., & Straurenghi, G. (2018). Optical coherence tomography angiography. *Prog Retin Eye Res*, 64, 1–55. https://doi.org/10.1016/j.preteyeres.2017.11.003.

Xu, D., Dávila, J. P., Rahimi, M., Rebhun, C. B., Alibhai, A. Y., Waheed, N. K., et al. (2018). Long-term progression of type 1 neovascularization in age-related macular degeneration using optical coherence tomography angiography. *American Journal of Ophthalmology*, 187, 10–20. https://doi.org/10.1016/j.ajo.2017.12.005.

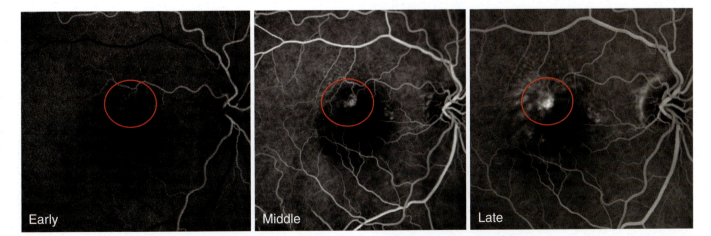

FIG. 6.2.1.1 Fluorescein angiography shows progressive hyperfluorescence, with dye accumulation within a fibrovascular pigment epithelial detachment surrounded by stippled fluorescence with unclear margins. This is the characteristic angiographic presentation of type 1 choroidal neovascularization.

*With contributions from Daniela Ferrara.

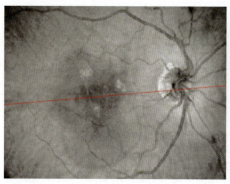 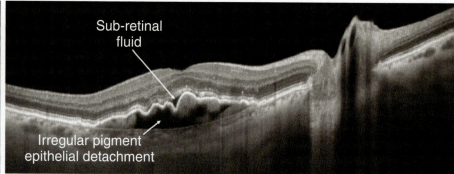

FIG. 6.2.1.2 OCT scan corresponding to the eye depicted in Fig. 6.2.1.1. The line scan shows an irregular pigment epithelial detachment (PED), which is characteristic of a type 1 choroidal neovascularization (CNV) lesion. The heterogeneous internal reflectivity of the PED and the presence of subretinal fluid also suggest this is an active (exudative) type 1 CNV.

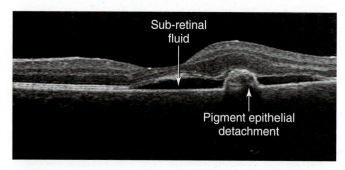 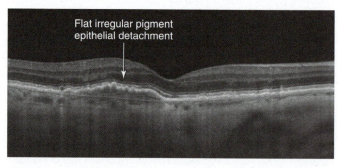

FIG. 6.2.1.3 OCT line scan shows a small pigment epithelial detachment with relatively heterogeneous internal reflectivity that is associated with subretinal fluid, characteristic of active (exudative) type 1 choroidal neovascularization.

FIG. 6.2.1.4 OCT line scan showing a flat, irregular pigment epithelial detachment (PED) characteristic of a type 1 choroidal neovascularization (CNV) lesion. Also seen is the stacked nature of the material within the CNV. Presence of fluid clefts within the PED (not present here) is very suggestive of an active type 1 lesion.

FIG. 6.2.1.5 OCT angiography en face and corresponding structural OCT B-scan showing a type 1 macular neovascularization (MNV) lesion. The cross hairs show that the lesion seen on the en face projection is a result of flow signal originating from beneath the retinal pigment epithelium and within the pigment epithelial detachment, indicative of a type 1 MNV membrane.

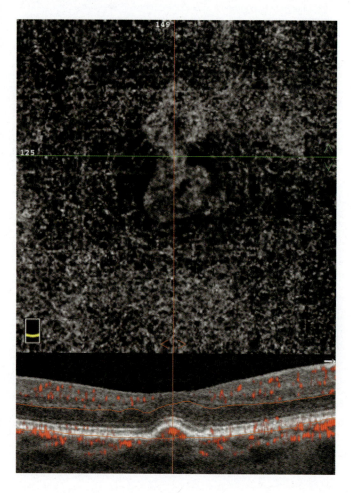

Type 2 Macular Neovascular Membrane

A. Yasin Alibhai

6.2.2

Summary

Type 2 macular neovascularization (MNV) extends through the subretinal space, between the neurosensory retina and the retinal pigment epithelium (RPE). It is characterized on fluorescein angiography as "classic choroidal neovascularization (CNV)," showing in the early phases of the angiogram the fine contour of the neovessels and in the late stages of the angiogram marked hyperfluorescence from profuse leakage (Fig. 6.2.2.1). On OCT, type 2 MNV typically manifests as subretinal hyperreflective material (Fig. 6.2.2.2) (Freund et al., 2010).

On OCT angiography (OCTA) imaging, type 2 MNVs appear as abnormal vessels in the normally "avascular" or deep retinal slab, with qualitative features similar to those of type 1 MNV membranes (Fig. 6.2.2.3) (Souied et al., 2016).

Type 2 MNV commonly occurs in association with exudative age-related macular degeneration (AMD) as well as in patients with acquired defects in their RPE–Bruch's membrane complex, such as pathologic myopia, retinochoroiditis, trauma, choroidal tumors, optic disc anomalies, and other primary conditions (Shah et al., 2014). These acquired defects provide a path of least resistance to the growth of abnormal blood vessels and serve as an entry point into the subretinal space. Depending on the cause, type 2 MNV can occur in association with type 1 MNV, forming a mixed neovascular complex. In this case, irregular pigment epithelial detachment (PED) with visible interruptions in the RPE layer are observed on OCT. Associated subretinal hemorrhage and subretinal fluid or intraretinal fluid may also be present (Fig. 6.2.2.4).

Key Points

- Type 2 MNV is classified based on its anatomic location, being present below the neurosensory retina but above the RPE.
- Type 2 MNV can be secondary to AMD or a result of acquired defects in the RPE–basement membrane complex, such as in pathologic myopia, retinochoroiditis, trauma, choroidal hamartomas, and optic disc anomalies.
- Depending on the cause, type 2 MNV can occur in association with type 1 MNV.

REFERENCES

Freund, K. B., Zweifel, S. A., & Engelbert, M. (2010). Do we need a new classification for choroidal neovascularization in age-related macular degeneration? *Retina, 30*(9), 1333–1349.

Shah, V. P., Shah, S. A., Mrejen, S., & Freund, K. B. (2014). Subretinal hyperreflective exudation associated with neovascular age-related macular degeneration. *Retina, 34*, 1281–1288.

Souied, E. H., El Ameen, A., Semoun, O., Miere, A., Querques, G., & Cohen, S. Y. (2016). Optical coherence tomography angiography of type 2 neovascularization in age-related macular degeneration. *Developments in Ophthalmology, 56*, 52–56.

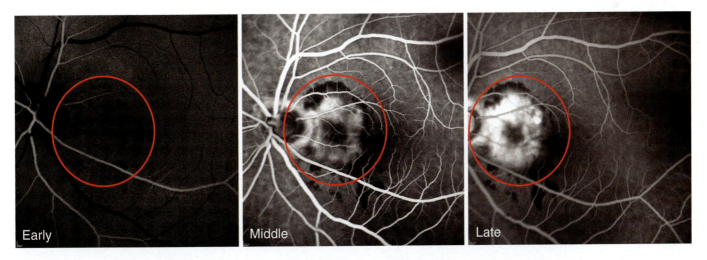

FIG. 6.2.2.1 Fluorescein angiography shows in the early phase of the angiogram, the fine contour of choroidal neovascularization (CNV) above the retinal pigment epithelium, and marked hyperfluorescence in the late phase secondary to profuse leakage typical of classic CNV.

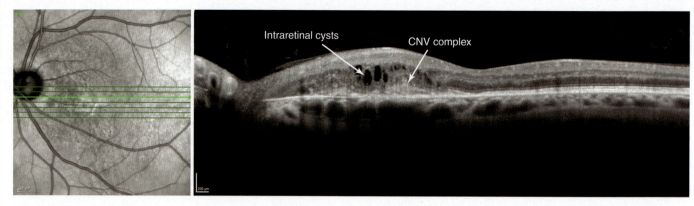

FIG. 6.2.2.2 OCT scan corresponding to the eye depicted in Fig. 6.2.2.1. There is subretinal hyperreflective material corresponding to the type 2 macular neovascularization complex located above split retinal pigment epithelium. Intraretinal cysts are also present.

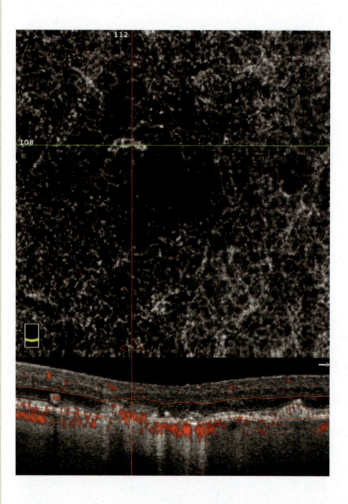

FIG. 6.2.2.3 OCT angiography en face and corresponding structural OCT B-scan showing a type 2 macular neovascularization (MNV) lesion. The cross hairs show that the lesion seen on the en face projection is a result of flow signal originating from above the retinal pigment epithelium, indicative of a type 2 MNV membrane. (Souied EH, El Ameen A, Semoun O, et al. Optical coherence tomography angiography of type 2 neovascularization in age-related macular degeneration. Dev Ophthalmol. 2016;56:52-6. Copyright © 2016, © 2016 S. Karger AG, Basel.)

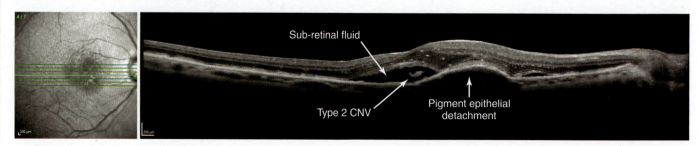

FIG. 6.2.2.4 OCT scan of a mixed macular neovascularization lesion showing the type 2 component. There is a pigment epithelial detachment with subretinal fluid.

Type 3 Macular Neovascular Membrane

A. Yasin Alibhai

Summary

Type 3 macular neovascularization (MNV) results from the proliferation of abnormal blood vessels from deep within the retinal tissue. These new intraretinal vessels are also known as retinal angiomatous proliferation (RAP) lesions. Type 3 MNV may grow within the neurosensory retina or down toward the choroid, forming chorioretinal anastomosis. Type 3 MNV typically occurs secondary to age-related macular degeneration (AMD), in eyes with confluent soft drusen (Fig. 6.2.3.1).

On OCT, the intraretinal neovascularization is typically associated with marked intraretinal fluid and intraretinal cystic changes, as well as occasionally with subretinal fluid (Fig. 6.2.3.2). Hyperreflective material below the neurosensory retinal also may be present. Chorioretinal anastomosis results in irregular pigment epithelial detachment (PED) (Fig. 6.2.3.3). On OCT angiography (OCTA), the retinal portion of type 3 MNVs can be observed as a distinct lesion with high flow signal, anastomosing with the choroidal vessels (Fig. 6.2.3.4) (Phasukkijwatana et al., 2017).

Type 3 MNVs are exquisitely responsive to anti–vascular endothelial growth factor (VEGF) agents. Very commonly, collapse of a PED may lead to atrophy.

Key Points

- Type 3 MNV corresponds to RAP. This MNV subtype originates within the retina and eventually evolves with chorioretinal anastomosis.
- Type 3 MNV is secondary to exudative AMD.
- On OCT, type 3 MNV is commonly associated with marked intraretinal fluid accumulation and subretinal fluid.
- On OCTA, type 3 MNV membranes can be seen extending from the middle retinal layers into the sub-RPE space.
- Atrophy of the RPE often develops upon collapse of an associated PED.

BIBLIOGRAPHY

Freund, K. B., Ho, I. V., Barbazetto, I. A., Koizumi, H., Laud, K., Ferrara, D., et al. (2008). Type 3 neovascularization: The expanded spectrum of retinal angiomatous proliferation. *Retina, 28*, 201–211.

Phasukkijwatana, N., Tan, A. C. S., Chen, X., Freund, K. B., & Sarraf, D. (2017). Optical coherence tomography angiography of type 3 neovascularisation in age-related macular degeneration after antiangiogenic therapy. *British Journal of Ophthalmology, 101*(5), 597–602.

Yannuzzi, L. A., Negrao, S., Iida, T., Carvalho, C., Rodriguez-Coleman, H., Slakter, J., et al. (2001). Retinal angiomatous proliferation in age-related macular degeneration. *Retina, 21*, 416–434.

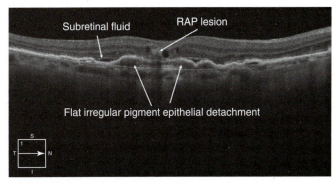

FIG. 6.2.3.2 OCT scan of a type 3 macular neovascularization lesion. There is an area of hyperreflectivity in the outer retina overlying the pigment epithelial detachment. Intraretinal cystic changes are also present. Reticular pseudodrusen are observed in the surrounding macular area. *RAP*, Retinal angiomatous proliferation.

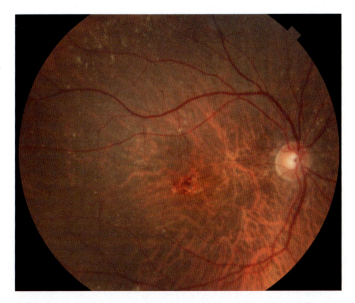

FIG. 6.2.3.1 Color fundus image of an eye with retinal angiomatous proliferation, or type 3 macular neovascularization, shows an area of subretinal hemorrhage. Reticular pseudodrusen are also present.

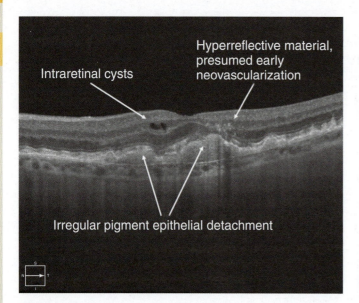

FIG. 6.2.3.3 OCT scan of a type 3 macular neovascularization lesion with hyperreflective material under the neurosensory retina.

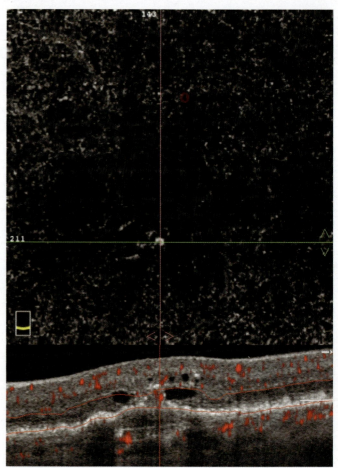

FIG. 6.2.3.4 OCT angiography en face and corresponding structural OCT b scan showing a Type 3 macular neovascularization (MNV) lesion. The cross hairs show that the lesion seen on the en face projection is a result of flow signal originating from within the retina, indicative of a type 3 MNV membrane. Associated intraretinal fluid and cystic changes are also present.

Summary

Subretinal hemorrhage (SRH) can be caused by various choroidal and retinal vascular abnormalities. However, the most common cause of those involving the macula is macular neovascularization (MNV), secondary to age-related macular degeneration (AMD). SRH can vary in size and distribution. The clinical appearance is that of a dark red area with normal overlying retinal vessels and fairly well-demarcated margins (Fig. 6.2.4.1). There may also be associated breakthrough intraretinal or vitreous hemorrhage. Large submacular hemorrhages tend to have a poorer prognosis regardless of any attempted intervention. Damage to the photoreceptors is a consequence of the toxic nature of blood and its components (iron, hemosiderin, and fibrin) within the subretinal spaces, sheer forces created by clot retraction, and physical separation from the retinal pigment epithelium (RPE) layer. This can result in atrophy and disciform scar formation regardless of treatment approach. On clinical examination or fundus photographs, it is challenging to differentiate SRH from sub-RPE hemorrhage, although the latter tends to be darker because of the overlying RPE.

On OCT, SRH appears as optically dense, hyperreflective material accumulated under the neurosensory retina (Fig. 6.2.4.2). Depending on the cause, it can be associated with additional changes—for example, pigment epithelial detachment secondary to type 1 MNV.

Key Points

- On OCT, SRH appears as hyperreflective material underneath the neurosensory retina.
- The most common cause of SRH is MNV secondary to AMD; other causes include myopia, trauma, angioid streaks, and histoplasmosis.
- The size of SRH can vary; larger hemorrhages carry a poorer visual prognosis.

BIBLIOGRAPHY

Bressler, N. M., Bressler, S. B., & Fine, S. L. (2006). (4th ed.). In S. P. (2006). Schachat Andrew (Ed.), *Neovascular (exudative) age-related macular degeneration in retina* (Vol. II). Mosby: Elsevier. Chapter 61.

*With contributions from Daniela Ferrara

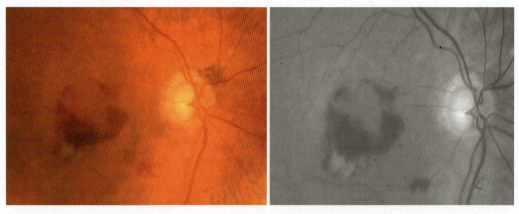

FIG. 6.2.4.1 Color fundus image and red-free image of subretinal hemorrhage. Note the dark color of the blood.

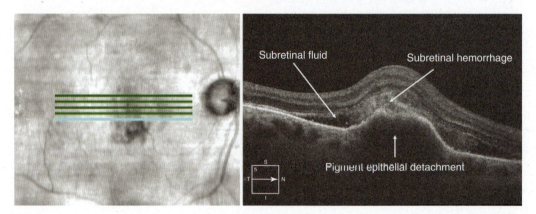

FIG. 6.2.4.2 OCT line scan corresponding to the eye depicted in Fig. 6.2.4.1 shows subretinal hemorrhage and subretinal fluid with an associated pigment epithelial detachment.

Summary

A disciform scar represents the end stage of a macular neovascularization (MNV) lesion. Fibrovascular tissue develops within Bruch's membrane, the subretinal space, and the subretinal pigment epithelium space. The retinal pigment epithelium (RPE) undergoes thickening in and around the area of scarring, and cystic degeneration of the overlying retina results in photoreceptor loss (Fig. 6.2.5.1). Although these scars are usually considered stable, disease activity may still persist in an adjacent MNV lesion, with recurring hemorrhage and exudation being the most common signs of activity.

On OCT, a disciform scar appears as hyperreflective tissue with distinct borders, underneath the neurosensory retina. Attenuation or complete loss of the outer retinal layers, especially the photoreceptor layer, is commonly seen above the disciform scar. Intraretinal cystic spaces can be present as a result of retinal degeneration (Fig. 6.2.5.2).

Key Points

- Disciform scar represents the end stage of MNV.
- It appears as hyperreflective subretinal material on OCT.

BIBLIOGRAPHY

Spaide, R. F. (2013). Clinical manifestations of choroidal neovascularization in AMD. In F. G. Holz, D. Pauleikhoff, R. F. Spaide, & A. C. Bird (Eds.), *Age-related macular degeneration* (3rd ed.). Berlin, Heidelberg: Springer Berlin Heidelberg.

FIG. 6.2.5.1 Color fundus photograph of a subretinal disciform scar from macular neovascularization secondary to age-related macular degeneration.

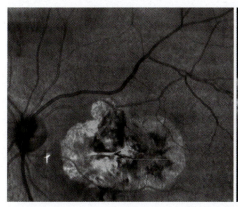
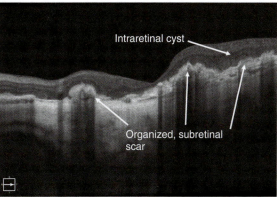

FIG. 6.2.5.2 Corresponding OCT scan of disciform scar seen in Fig. 6.2.5.1. Hyperreflective material is present in the subretinal space that corresponds to the organized subretinal scar. Note loss of the photoreceptor layer above the scar and degenerative intraretinal cystic changes not associated with macular neovascularization activity. Shadowing underlies the scar.

*With contributions from Daniela Ferrara

Summary

Retinal pigment epithelium (RPE) tears develop because of pigment epithelial detachments (PEDs) secondary to macular neovascularization (MNV), retinal angiomatous proliferation (RAP) lesions, or polypoidal choroidal vasculopathy (PCV). They can occur without treatment for MNV or after thermal laser, photodynamic therapy, or anti–vascular endothelial growth factor (VEGF) therapy. The mechanisms behind an RPE tear are thought to be the result of two opposing forces: traction from MNV contraction and adhesion from the RPE that is still attached. An RPE tear involving the fovea usually results in a devastating visual outcome; therefore, prognostic markers that are predictive of RPE tear formation have been investigated. Studies have shown that PEDs measuring more than 400 µm in height have a higher risk for evolving into RPE tears.

On OCT, RPE tears appear as hyperreflective tissue rolled up underneath the neurosensory retina, with a free edge of "wavy" RPE at the margins of an area with exposed Bruch's membrane and absent overlying RPE (Fig. 6.2.6.1). The outer neurosensory retinal layers may have normal appearance or may be thinned.

Key Points

- RPE tears develop because of PED secondary to MNV.
- On OCT, RPE tears appear as hyperreflective tissue rolled up underneath the neurosensory retina and adjacent to an area with complete RPE loss.

BIBLIOGRAPHY

Chan, C. K., Abraham, P., Meyer, C. H., Kokami, G. T., Kaiser, P. K., Rauser, M. E., et al. (2010). Optical coherence tomography-measured pigment epithelial detachment height as a predictor for retinal pigment epithelial tears associated with intravitreal bevacizumab injections. *Retina, 30*, 203–211.

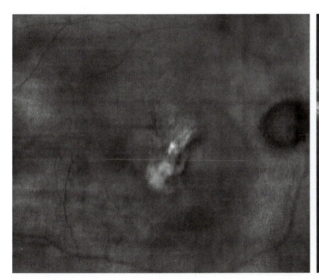
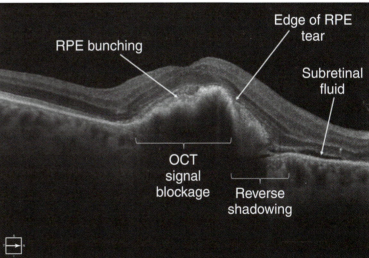

FIG. 6.2.6.1 OCT line scan through an area of retinal hemorrhage shows a retinal pigment epithelium (*RPE*) tear. The absence of the RPE in the region of the tear allows for deeper penetration of the OCT signal, creating the characteristic "reverse shadowing" (or "hypertransmission") sign. The RPE is rolled up where it is still present, resulting in OCT signal blockage and reduced visibility of deeper structures.

*With contributions from Daniela Ferrara

A. Yasin Alibhai*

Summary

Polypoidal choroidal vasculopathy (PCV) manifests as a variant of type 1 macular neovascularization (MNV), more commonly occurring in African-American or Asian individuals. Its cause is still not fully understood, and many authors consider it as a variant of age-related macular degeneration (AMD). However, it can present itself as a distinct clinical entity, without the typical clinical features of AMD or in conjunction with typical clinical findings (drusen, pigmentary changes) (Fig. 6.2.7.1). PCV lesions are characterized by polyp-shaped vascular complexes located beneath the retinal pigment epithelium (RPE) layer.

Typical OCT findings include multiple large pigment epithelial detachments (PEDs) with associated subretinal fluid. These PEDs may have, adherent to their posterior surface, round-oval cavities with hyperreflective borders representing the polypoidal lesions (Fig. 6.2.7.2). Exudate due to PCV lesions appear as hyperreflective intraretinal spots visible on OCT line scans. Often, a large PED is adjacent to a smaller, flat PED or adjacent to elevated RPE with underlying moderately hyperreflective tissue, representing the branching vascular network that is thought to feed the polyps (Fig. 6.2.7.3). Subretinal hyperreflective material may also be observed in some cases. En face structural OCT is particularly useful in supporting the diagnosis of PCV and documenting the entire extent of the lesion. OCT angiography may demonstrate the branching vascular network in PCV lesions (Fig. 6.2.7.4). However, studies have shown a varying degree of sensitivity in detecting polyps using OCT angiography (OCTA) due to possible variations in blood flow speeds within the neovascular complex. In challenging or atypical cases, multimodal imaging might be helpful in the differential diagnosis of PCV, especially indocyanine-green angiography (ICGA) (Fig. 6.2.7.5).

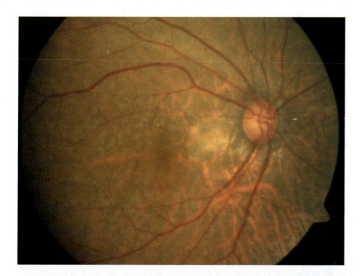

FIG. 6.2.7.1 Color fundus photograph of an eye with a peripapillary polypoidal choroidal vasculopathy lesion that has subretinal fluid accumulation. Reticular pseudodrusen are also observed.

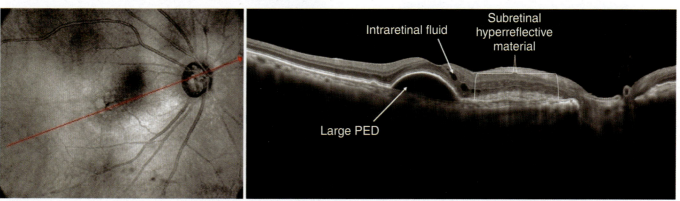

Intraretinal fluid

Subretinal hyperreflective material

Large PED

FIG. 6.2.7.2 OCT line scan corresponding to Fig. 6.2.7.1. The OCT shows a large pigment epithelial detachment *(PED)* with internal hyporeflectivity adjacent to a flat PED with heterogeneous internal hyperreflectivity where a vascular lumen is observed. Overlying intraretinal fluid is present, and subretinal hyperreflective material is associated with the PED.

*With contributions from Daniela Ferrara

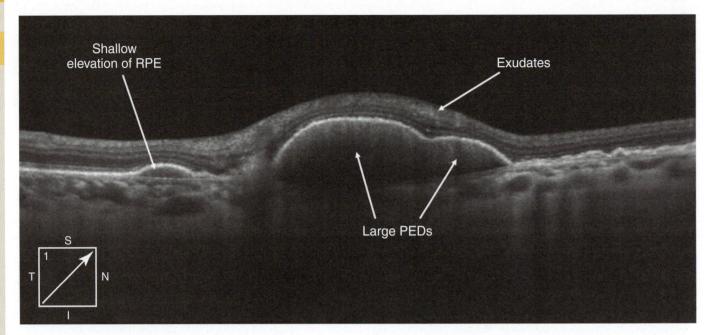

FIG. 6.2.7.3 OCT line scan shows multiple large PEDs adjacent to a shallow PED. The branching vascular network typically lies within the shallow RPE elevation and supplies the polyps beneath the large PEDs. *PED*, Pigment epithelial detachment; *RPE*, retinal pigment epithelium.

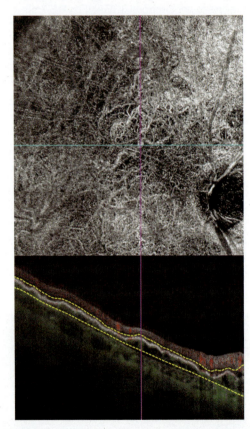

FIG. 6.2.7.4 OCT angiography en face and corresponding structural OCT B-scan of an eye with a polypoidal choroidal vasculopathy lesion. The cross hairs on the en face projection are centered on a polyp with a corresponding branching vascular network visible. The structural OCT B-scan shows a shallow pigment epithelial detachment with flow signal within, corresponding to the visible polyp.

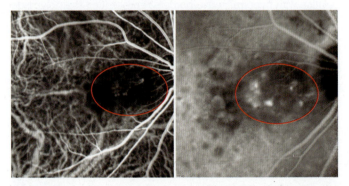

FIG. 6.2.7.5 Indocyanine-green angiography corresponding to the eye depicted in Fig. 6.2.7.1. Early phase image *(left)* shows a branching vascular network *(red circle)*, and late frame image shows hyperfluorescent polyps consistent with the diagnosis of polypoidal choroidal vasculopathy.

Key Points

- PCV presents a variant of type 1 MNV.
- OCT findings typical of PCV lesions include multiple large PEDs.
- Round-oval polyps may be adherent to the posterior surface of associated PED.
- A branching vascular network may be seen underlying a flat PED adjacent to the polyp, which is particularly well visualized on en face structural OCT.
- OCT angiography identifies polyps in some, but not all, PCV lesions, likely due to variable blood flow speeds within the polyp.

BIBLIOGRAPHY

Alasil, T., Ferrara, D., Adhi, M., Brewer, E., Kraus, M. F., Baumal, C. R., et al. (2015). En face imaging of the choroid in polypoidal choroidal vasculopathy using swept-source optical coherence tomography. *American Journal of Ophthalmology*, *159*(4), 634–643. https://doi.org/10.1016/j.ajo.2014.12.012.

Rebhun, C., Moult, E., Novais, E., Moreira-Neto, C., Ploner, S. B., Louzada, R. M., et al. (2017). Polypoidal choroidal vasculopathy on swept-source optical coherence tomography angiography with variable interscan time analysis. *Translations Vision Science & Technology*, *6*(6), 4.

Yannuzzi, L. A., Sorenson, J., Spaide, R. F., Lipson, B. (1990). Idiopathic polypoidal choroidal vasculopathy (IPCV). *Retina*, *10*, 1–8.

Vitreomacular Adhesion

Darin R. Goldman

7.1

Summary

During the normal evolution of age-related vitreomacular separation, areas of vitreous may remain attached to the macula (see Chapter 27.1). Vitreomacular adhesion represents a normal physiologic state of the vitreomacular interface (Fig. 7.1.1). The degree of adhesion can vary from focal to broad (Figs. 7.1.2 and 7.1.3). This benign finding is distinguished from the pathologic state of vitreomacular traction (see Chapter 7.2) as a result of the lack of distortion or disruption of the retinal layers and no impact on vision. The presence of vitreomacular adhesion can be helpful to determine future risk for vitreomacular interface disorders.

Key OCT Features

- Vitreomacular adhesion may be focal or broad.
- Vitreomacular adhesion is a benign physiologic finding (Fig. 7.1.4) that should be distinguished from similar, often pathologic, states of the vitreomacular interface.
- In a patient with a history of full-thickness macular hole (FTMH) in one eye, if vitreomacular adhesion is present in the fellow eye, there is a risk for future FTMH formation in that eye.

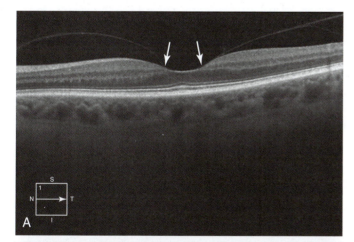

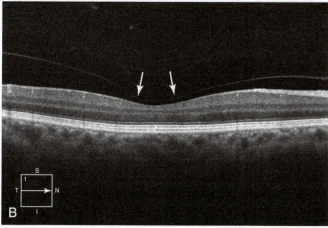

FIG. 7.1.1 (A and B) Focal vitreomacular adhesion is present overlying the central macula. The posterior hyaloid is seen inserting near the edges of the fovea *(arrows)* without any disturbance of the normal foveal contour.

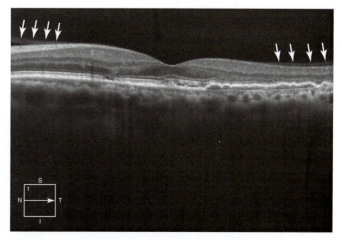

FIG. 7.1.2 Broad vitreomacular adhesion is present over the entire macula. The posterior face of the hyaloid blends, almost imperceptibly, with the surface of the macula *(arrows)*. This eye later developed vitreomacular traction with an FTMH.

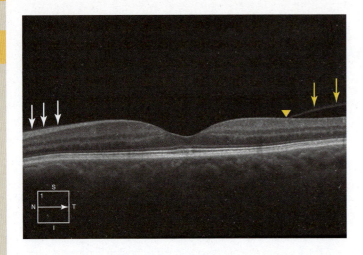

FIG. 7.1.3 Broad vitreomacular adhesion beginning to release. Nasally, the posterior hyaloid is still adherent to the macular surface *(white arrows)*. Temporally, the posterior hyaloid has begun to release from the macula at a focal point *(yellow arrowhead)*, beyond where there is release of the adhesion *(yellow arrows)*.

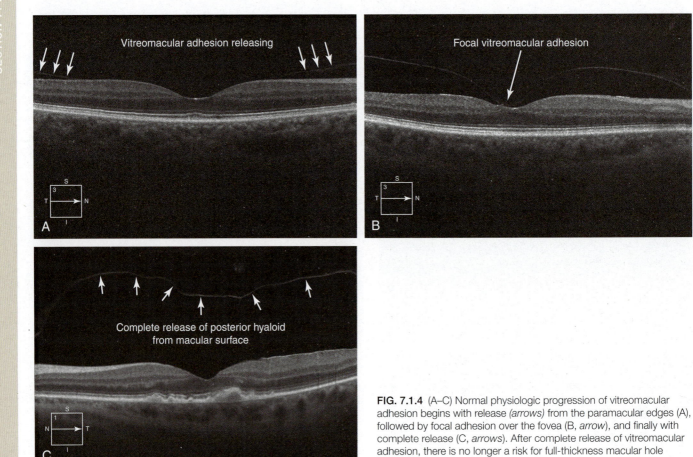

FIG. 7.1.4 (A–C) Normal physiologic progression of vitreomacular adhesion begins with release *(arrows)* from the paramacular edges (A), followed by focal adhesion over the fovea (B, *arrow*), and finally with complete release (C, *arrows*). After complete release of vitreomacular adhesion, there is no longer a risk for full-thickness macular hole development.

Summary

Vitreomacular traction (VMT) syndrome falls into the broad category of vitreomacular interface disorders. VMT occurs when the posterior hyaloid fails to separate normally from the central macular surface during abnormal posterior vitreous detachment (Figs. 7.2.1–7.2.7). The degree of traction over the fovea varies from a pinpoint spot to a broad area. Secondary effects on the macula include distortion of retinal layers, cystoid macular edema, and subretinal fluid (Fig. 7.2.6). Visual impairment can vary from mild to severe. VMT often will release spontaneously; therefore, an initial period of observation is usually warranted. However, VMT also may worsen or progress to a lamellar hole or full-thickness macular hole (FTMH) (Figs. 7.2.4 and 7.2.5). Pharmacologic or surgical interventions should be considered if symptoms become significantly bothersome to the patient.

Key OCT Features

- VMT is due to an abnormally strong focal adhesion of the posterior hyaloid to the macula.
- VMT is distinguished on OCT by disruption of the normal macular contour at a focal point with overlying vitreous insertion.
- VMT may resolve spontaneously or progress to visually impactful sequela, including lamellar macular hole and FTMH.

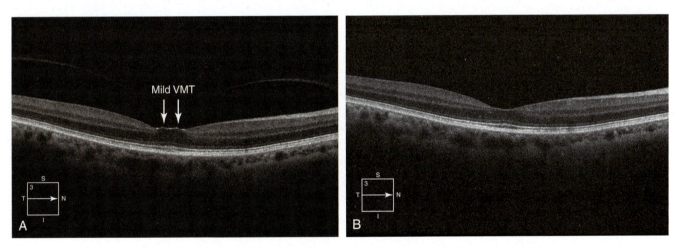

FIG. 7.2.1 (A and B) Mild vitreomacular traction (A) spontaneously releases over time, leaving a normal macular contour (B).

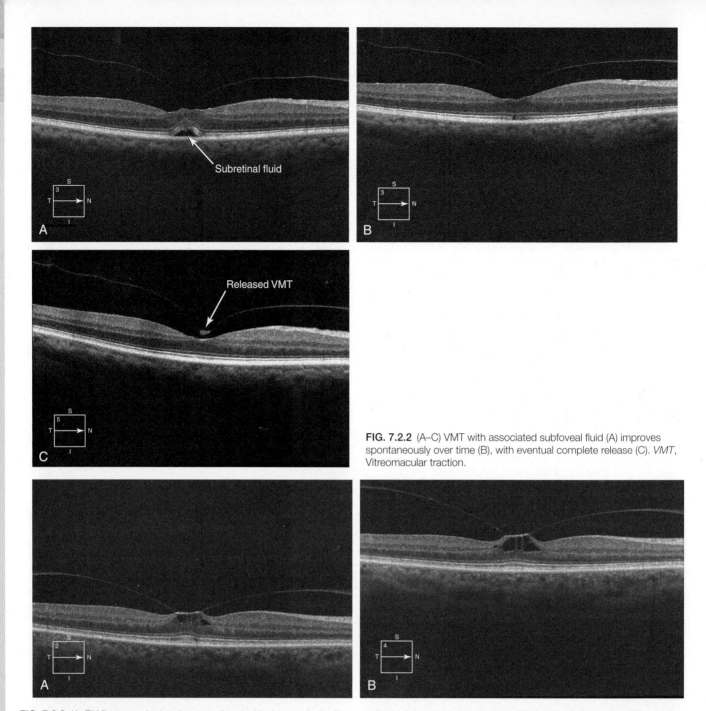

FIG. 7.2.2 (A–C) VMT with associated subfoveal fluid (A) improves spontaneously over time (B), with eventual complete release (C). *VMT*, Vitreomacular traction.

FIG. 7.2.3 (A–B) Vitreomacular traction associated with changes in the fovea similar to those in tractional schisis (A) that worsen over time (B). Intervention may be considered, depending on the visual impact.

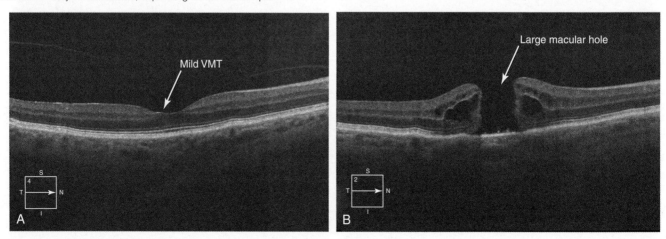

FIG. 7.2.4 (A and B) Mild VMT (A) may progress to a large full-thickness macular hole over time (B). This evolution was not possible to predict. *VMT*, Vitreomacular traction.

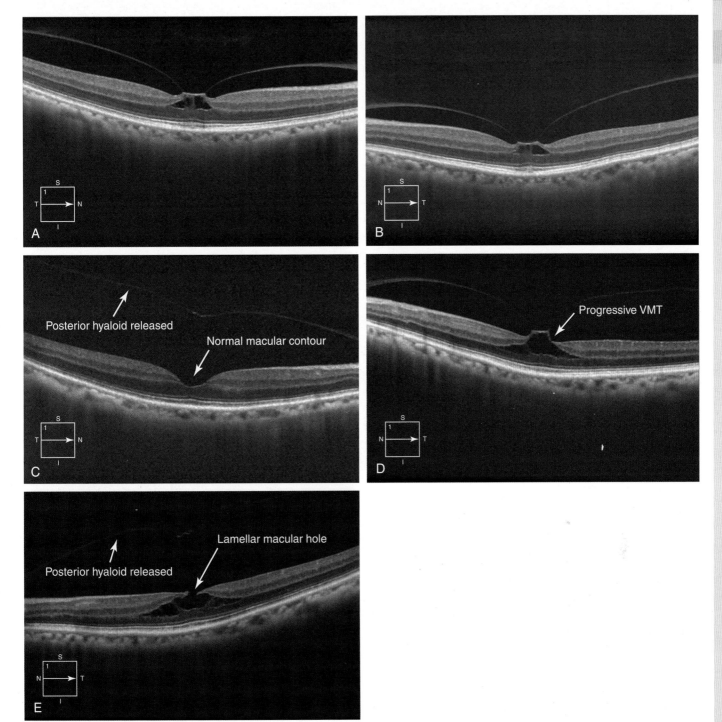

FIG. 7.2.5 (A–E) VMT present in both eyes (A and B). With release of the posterior hyaloid from the macular surface, spontaneous normalization of the macular contour (C) or development of a lamellar macular hole (D and E) can occur. *VMT*, Vitreomacular traction

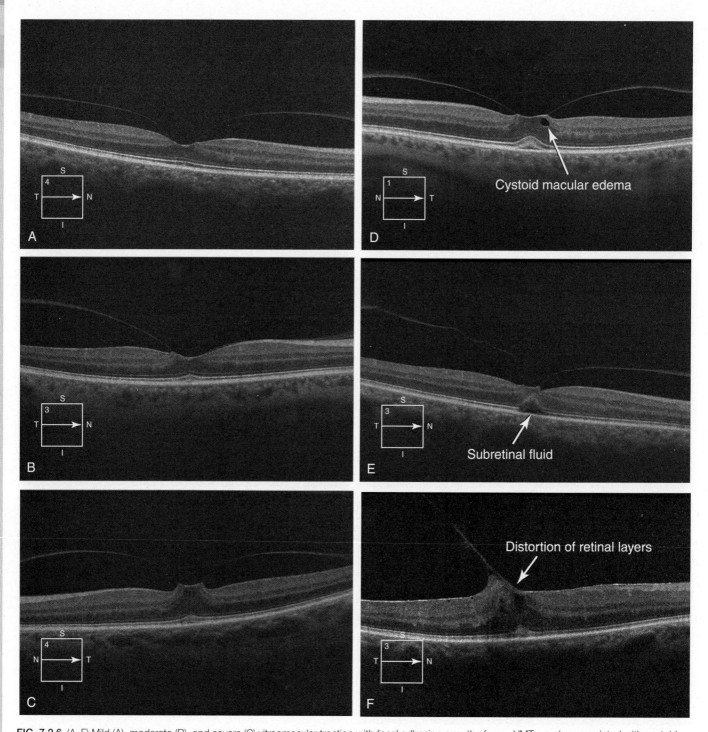

FIG. 7.2.6 (A–F) Mild (A), moderate (B), and severe (C) vitreomacular traction with focal adhesion over the fovea. VMT may be associated with cystoid macular edema (D), subretinal fluid (E), and distortion of the retinal layers (F).

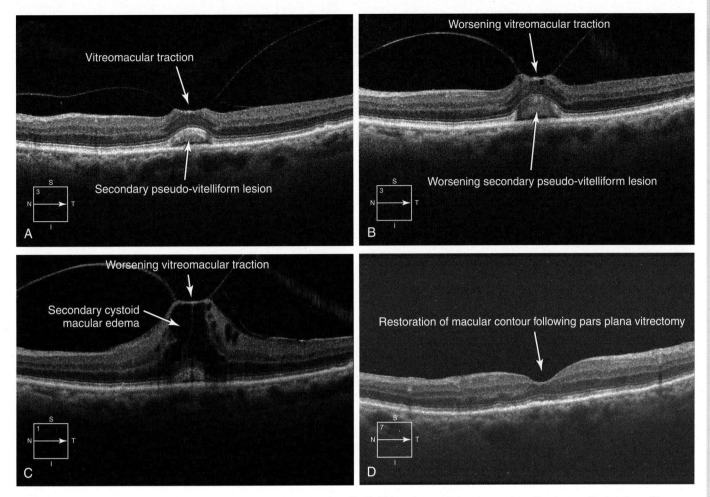

FIG. 7.2.7 (A–D) Vitreomacular traction may significantly worsen over time (A–C). This patient underwent pars plana vitrectomy with elevation of the hyaloid; postoperatively the patient experienced a dramatic normalization of the macular contour and a significant improvement in visual acuity (D).

Summary

Normally, with aging, there is progressive liquefaction of the vitreous body and eventual complete separation of the posterior hyaloid from the macula during posterior vitreous detachment. Full-thickness macular holes (FTMHs) typically develop in a predisposed individual who has an abnormally taut adhesion between the vitreous and the central macula (Figs. 7.3.1–7.3.8). In these persons, during posterior vitreous detachment evolution, focal traction on the fovea results in the development of a full-thickness defect or hole. FTMHs are described based on diameter and the presence or absence of vitreomacular traction (VMT) according to the International Vitreomacular Traction Study Classification System (Duker et al., 2013).

Key Points

- Small FTMHs have a diameter of 250 µm or less (Figs. 7.3.1–7.3.3).
- Medium FTMHs have a diameter between 250 and 400 µm Fig. 7.3.4.
- Large FTMHs have a diameter greater than 400 µm Figs. 7.3.5–7.3.6.
- The presence or absence of VMT is important in classifying FTMHs.
- The size of an FTMH is determined based on the minimum hole width at the narrowest point in the midretina (Figs. 7.3.1, 7.3.4, and 7.3.5).

REFERENCE

Duker, J. S., Kaiser, P. K., Binder, S., de Smet, M. D., Gaudruic, A., Reichel, E., et al. (2013). The International Vitreomacular Traction Study Group classification of vitreomacular adhesion, traction, and macular hole. *Ophthalmology*, *120*(12), 2611–2619.

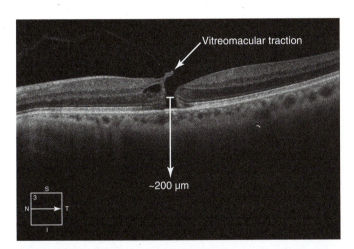

FIG. 7.3.1 A small full-thickness macular hole (~200 µm diameter) with vitreomacular traction.

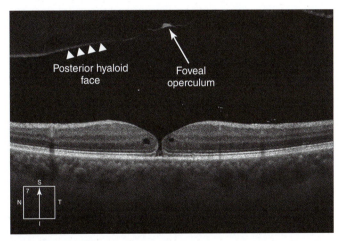

FIG. 7.3.3 A small full-thickness macular hole without vitreomacular traction. The posterior hyaloid face and a foveal operculum are visible toward the *top* of the image.

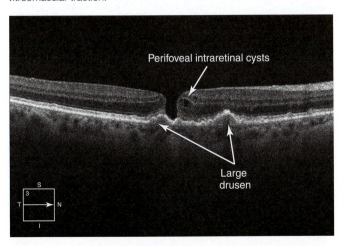

FIG. 7.3.2 A small full-thickness macular hole without vitreomacular traction. There are minimal perifoveal intraretinal cysts, the paucity of which suggests this hole is of more chronic duration. Incidentally, large drusen are present.

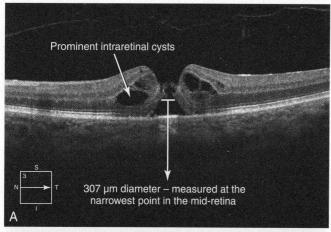

Prominent intraretinal cysts

307 µm diameter – measured at the narrowest point in the mid-retina

A

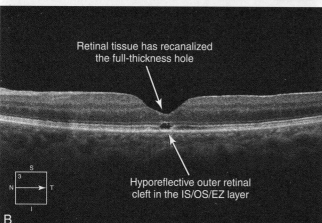

Retinal tissue has recanalized the full-thickness hole

Hyporeflective outer retinal cleft in the IS/OS/EZ layer

B

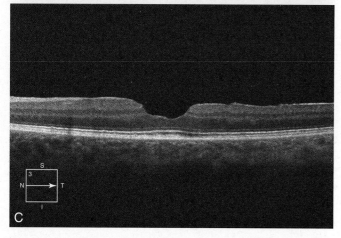

C

FIG. 7.3.4 (A) Medium full-thickness macular hole without vitreomacular traction. This image provides a good example of the proper location to measure the aperture of a macular hole—the minimum hole width at the narrowest point in the midretina. Prominent intraretinal cysts on the hole edge suggest that this hole is of relatively acute onset. (B) Typical appearance 2 weeks after pars plana vitrectomy with internal limiting membrane peeling and gas tamponade (corresponding to A). The foveal depression has returned; however, a hyporeflective outer retinal cavity is present. (C) Typical appearance 6 months postoperatively in which the foveal contour is well defined, although still somewhat irregular, and the outer retinal layers have fully returned and are continuous. *EZ*, Ellipsoid zone; *IS*, inner segments; *OS*, outer segments.

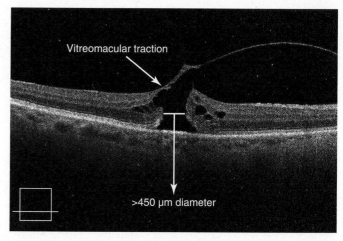

Vitreomacular traction

>450 µm diameter

FIG. 7.3.5 A large full-thickness macular hole with vitreomacular traction.

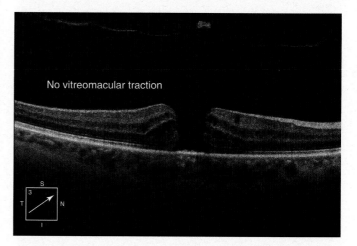

No vitreomacular traction

FIG. 7.3.6 A large full-thickness macular hole without vitreomacular traction.

Macula Thickness: Macular Cube 512 × 128   OD ● | ○ OS

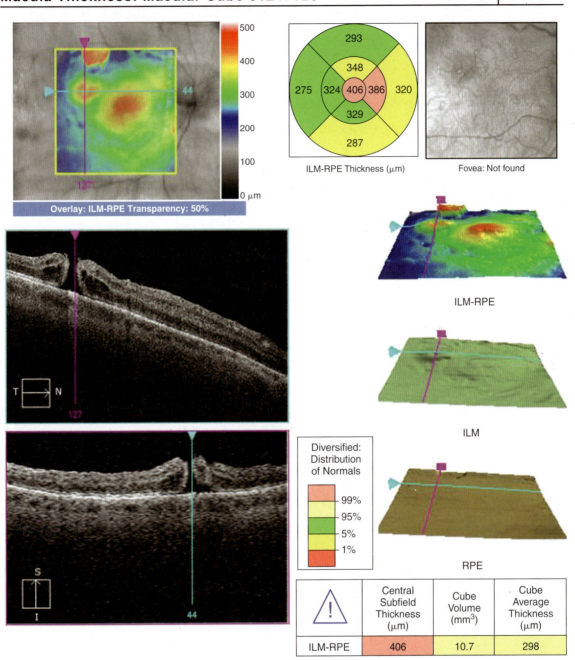

ILM-RPE Thickness (µm)

Fovea: Not found

Overlay: ILM-RPE Transparency: 50%

ILM-RPE

ILM

RPE

Diversified: Distribution of Normals

	99%
	95%
	5%
	1%

⚠	Central Subfield Thickness (µm)	Cube Volume (mm³)	Cube Average Thickness (µm)
ILM-RPE	406	10.7	298

FIG. 7.3.7 A volumetric map illustrates an eccentric full-thickness macular hole superotemporal to the fovea. This was noted in a patient after uneventful pars plana vitrectomy and membrane peeling for an epiretinal membrane, presumably iatrogenic. No additional treatment was performed, the patient was asymptomatic, and the hole remained stable over an extended period. *ILM,* Inner limiting membrane; *RPE,* retinal pigment epithelium.

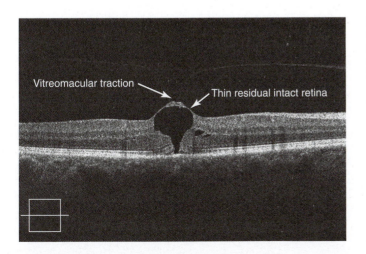

Vitreomacular traction
Thin residual intact retina

FIG. 7.3.8 This vitreomacular abnormality fits somewhere between vitreomacular traction (VMT) and an early full-thickness macular hole. A layer of inner retina is clearly still intact, but with time this would be expected to progress to a full-thickness defect. This case helps illustrate the dynamic nature of VMT and macular holes.

Summary

A lamellar macular hole or defect results from a variety of causes, such as abortive full-thickness macular hole (FTMH) or epiretinal membrane (ERM) formation that causes partial-thickness loss of the inner macular layers involving the fovea. Historically, this was an ill-defined clinical diagnosis; it has become more clearly defined with OCT. The characteristic appearance on OCT is an irregular, anvil-shaped inner foveal defect without loss of the outer retinal layers (Figs. 7.4.1–7.4.4). Schisis-like changes also may be seen between the inner and outer retinal layers. Associated ERMs are common. Lamellar macular hole can be distinguished from "macular pseudohole" in that there is no loss of foveal tissue in the latter (see Chapter 7.5). Visual acuity generally remains good.

Key OCT Features

- Foveal OCT features of lamellar macular hole include the following (Witkin et al., 2006):
  - Irregular foveal contour
  - Defect of inner fovea
  - Separation of the inner and outer retinal layers
  - Lack of a full-thickness retinal defect
- Lamellar macular holes typically remain stable over time, and surgical treatment is rarely required.

REFERENCE

Witkin, A. J., Ko, T. H., Fujimoto, J. G., Schuman, J. S., Baumal, C. R., Rogers, A. H., et al. (2006). Redefining lamellar holes and the vitreomacular interface: An ultrahigh-resolution optical coherence tomography study. *Ophthalmology*, *113*(3), 388–397.

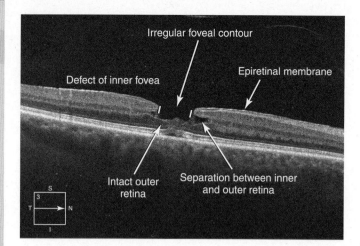

FIG. 7.4.1 Common features of lamellar macular hole are depicted, including an irregular foveal contour, a defect of the inner fovea (between bars), a separation between the inner and outer retina, and an intact outer retina (lack of full-thickness hole). There is also an associated ERM present, which is common.

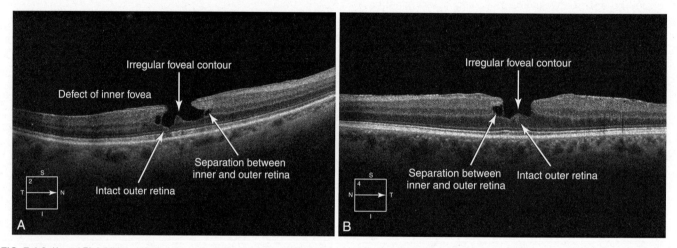

FIG. 7.4.2 (A and B) Additional typical examples of lamellar macular hole, depicting features similar to those in Fig. 7.4.1.

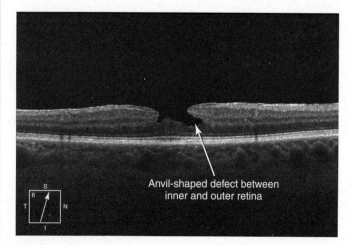

FIG. 7.4.3 In a lamellar macular hole, the defect between the inner and outer retina often conforms to an anvil shape. This area also may have schisis-like clefts.

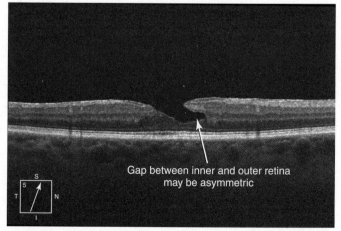

FIG. 7.4.4 Depending on the exact cross-section imaged, the defect between the inner and outer retina in a lamellar macular hole may be asymmetric.

Summary

Epiretinal membrane (ERM) formation is much more common than either vitreomacular traction (VMT) or lamellar macular hole formation, with a prevalence greater than 30% (Meuer et al., 2015). ERM may occur secondary to a variety of ocular conditions, such as uveitis, retinal tear, and retinal detachment. However, frequently, they are idiopathic with no identifiable cause. In these cases, in which a posterior vitreous detachment is usually present, it is thought that residual posterior hyaloid forms a scaffold for the proliferation of cellular material on the surface of the macula. An ERM appears as a thin, hyperreflective sheet overlying the internal limiting membrane (Figs. 7.5.1–7.5.6). A mild ERM may cause little or no distortion of the underlying retinal layers and no impact on vision. With more severe proliferation, the macular contour can be quite disturbed, with loss of the foveal depression and resultant impairment in visual acuity (Fig. 7.5.7). Associated visual symptoms may include metamorphopsia, decreased visual acuity, micropsia, and monocular diplopia. Most cases are mild and do not require treatment. More severe cases with visual impairment may require surgical removal.

Key OCT Features

- OCT is very sensitive in detecting the presence of an ERM, which appears as a hyperreflective, thickened membrane on the inner surface of the macula.
- An ERM may take on a corrugated or undulating contour in cross-section.
- In the presence of ERM, the macular contour may appear normal or become highly disorganized on OCT.

REFERENCE

Meuer, S. M., Myers, C. E., Klein, B. E., Swift, M. K., Huang, Y., Gangaputra, S., et al. (2015). The epidemiology of vitreoretinal interface abnormalities as detected by spectral-domain optical coherence tomography: The Beaver Dam Eye Study. *Ophthalmology*, *122*(4), 787–795.

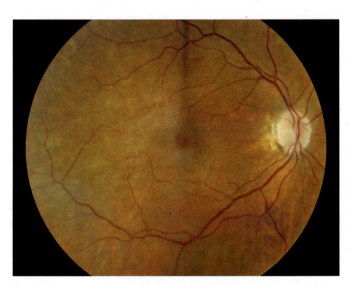

FIG. 7.5.1 Color photograph showing a typical macular appearance of an epiretinal membrane with irregular sheen, loss of the foveal reflex, and distortion of the normal vascular pattern.

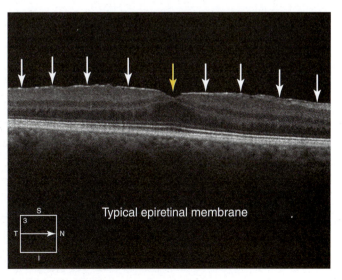

FIG. 7.5.2 Typical OCT appearance of epiretinal membrane showing a hyperreflective, thin membrane overlying the surface of the macula. The normal smooth contour of the macula is replaced by corrugations of the macular surface *(white arrows)*. There is loss of the foveal depression *(yellow arrow)*.

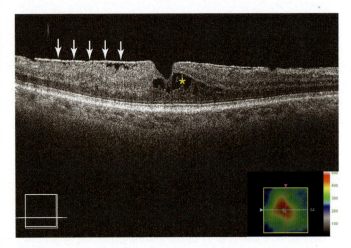

FIG. 7.5.3 Typical epiretinal membrane appearance *(white arrows)*. Associated schisis-like changes are present between the inner and outer retina *(asterisk)*, similar to the appearance of a lamellar macular hole. The corresponding thickness map *(inset)* shows thickening of the central macula in an irregular shape.

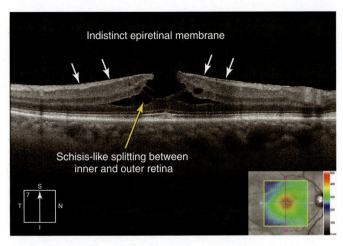

FIG. 7.5.4 The epiretinal membrane is somewhat indistinct *(white arrows)* and is associated with significant schisis between the inner and outer retinal layers, an apparent tractional effect. This could be considered a lamellar macular hole by some classification schemes.

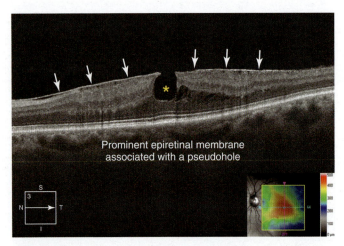

FIG. 7.5.5 A prominent epiretinal membrane *(arrows)* is associated with a pseudohole *(asterisk)*. No loss of retinal tissue occurred, which distinguishes this entity from a lamellar macular hole.

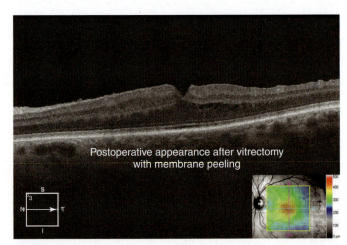

FIG. 7.5.6 Postoperative appearance after vitrectomy, with peeling of the epiretinal membrane corresponding to preoperative Fig. 7.5.5.

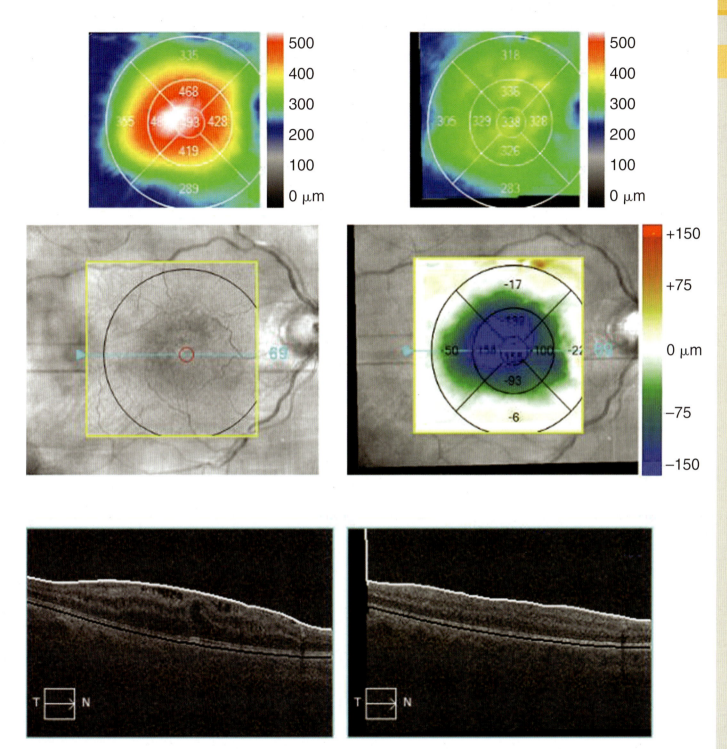

FIG. 7.5.7 In addition to B-scans, thickness and difference maps can be very illustrative in depicting changes over time, although correct segmentation is imperative. A typical epiretinal membrane shown preoperatively *(left)* and postoperatively after vitrectomy with membrane peeling *(right)*. The thickness maps *(top)* show normalization of macular thickness within the central macula. The difference map *(middle, right)* shows the corresponding degree of reduced thickness. Corresponding B-scans are also shown *(bottom)*.

Central Serous Chorioretinopathy

Eduardo A. Novais | Luiz Roisman

8.1

Summary

Central serous chorioretinopathy (CSCR) is a disease characterized by the serous detachment of the neurosensory retina that occurs over an area of leakage from the choriocapillaris through the retinal pigment epithelium (RPE) (Hussain & Gass, 1998; Wang et al., 2008; Yap & Robertson, 1996). Its frequency is around 10 cases per 100,000 and is sixfold higher in men than in women (Hussain & Gass, 1998; Wang et al., 2008; Yap & Robertson, 1996). The age at first diagnosis usually ranges from the third to the fifth decade (Hussain & Gass, 1998; Wang et al., 2008; Yap & Robertson, 1996). The pathophysiology is unknown; however, the most accepted theory claims that initial choroidal vascular hyperpermeability leads to secondary dysfunction of the overlying RPE (Hussain & Gass, 1998; Wang et al., 2008; Yap & Robertson, 1996). Type A personalities, exogenous steroid use, and systemic hypertension are the most common associations with the development of CSCR (Hussain & Gass, 1998; Wang et al., 2008; Yap & Robertson, 1996). Serous retinal detachments usually resolve spontaneously in most patients, and around 80%–90% return to 20/25 or better vision (Hussain & Gass, 1998; Wang et al., 2008; Yap & Robertson, 1996). A subset of patients may have recurrent or chronic serous retinal detachments, resulting in progressive RPE atrophy and permanent visual loss of 20/200 or worse. Macular neovascularization (MNV) may also develop in recurrent or chronic cases (Hussain & Gass, 1998; Wang et al., 2008; Yap & Robertson, 1996). Fluorescein angiography (FA) is currently considered the gold standard for diagnosis, and findings vary from discrete areas of focal leakage to diffuse RPE defect (Hussain & Gass, 1998; Wang et al., 2008; Yap & Robertson, 1996). However, in the last decade, OCT has played an important role in the diagnosis, prognosis, and follow-up of CSCR (Iida et al., 2000; Piccolino et al., 2005; Yang et al., 2013). It can demonstrate some typical features of CSCR, such as choroidal thickening, subretinal fluid, and pigmented epithelium detachment (PED). Choroidal thickening is a key feature on CSCR, and Agrawal et al. (2016) showed that this thickening is caused by an increase in vascular tissue or lumen, not by interstitial tissue, which corroborates the hypothesis of choroidal vascular congestion. Subretinal fluid is typically macular, although extramacular foci may be found. Commonly, PED in CSCR has a semicircular shape with hyporeflective content and can vary in height (Song et al., 2012). Recently, the terminology "shallow irregular RPE elevation" (SIRE) has been used to describe a PED that may correspond to MNV. It was recently reported and is a more elaborately defined term of the widely used concept "double-layer sign," previously described by Sato et al. (de Oliveira Dias et al., 2018; Narita et al., 2020; Sato et al., 2007). SIRE is defined as RPE elevations with a greatest transverse linear dimension of 1000 µm or more, a shallow (height of less than 100 µm) and irregular RPE layer, and a heterogeneous internal reflectivity. A microrip of the RPE or fissure is defined as a small breach in the RPE and is usually located within the areas of hyperfluorescence on the indocyanine-green angiography (ICGA) images (Ranjan et al., 2020; Yang et al., 2013).

OCT angiography is an important imaging modality that may be able to visualize flow impairment of the choriocapillaris and, most importantly, play a role in the early detection of secondary MNV (Feucht et al., 2016; Shinojima et al., 2016).

OCT Key Findings

- Serous macular detachment (Fig. 8.1.1).
- RPE detachment (Fig. 8.1.2).
- Choroidal thickening (Fig. 8.1.3).
- Outer retina granulations (Fig. 8.1.4).
- SIRE (Fig. 8.1.5B).
- Choroidal neovascularization seen on OCT angiography (Fig. 8.1.5D).
- RPE microrip (Fig. 8.1.6).

REFERENCES

Agrawal, R., Chhablani, J., Tan, K. -A., Shah, S., Sarvaiya, C., & Banker, A. (2016). Choroidal vascularity index in central serous chorioretinopathy. *Retina*, 36, 1646–1651.

de Oliveira Dias, J. R., Zheng, F., Motulsky, E. H., Roisman, L., Miller, A., Chen, C, -L., et al. (2018). Natural history of subclinical neovascularization in nonexudative age-related macular degeneration using swept-source OCT angiography. *Ophthalmology*, 125, 255–266.

Feucht, N., Maier, M., Lohmann, C. P., & Reznicek, L. (2016). OCT angiography findings in acute central serous chorioretinopathy. *Ophthalmic Surgery, Lasers, & Imaging Retina*, 47, 322–327.

Hussain, D., & Gass, J. D. (1998). Idiopathic central serous chorioretinopathy. *Indian Journal of Ophthalmology*, 46, 131–137.

Iida, T., Hagimura, N., Sato, T., & Kishi, S. (2000). Evaluation of central serous chorioretinopathy with optical coherence tomography. *American Journal of Ophthalmology*, 129, 16–20.

Narita, C., Hagimura, N., Sato, T., & Kishi, S. (2020). Structural OCT signs suggestive of subclinical nonexudative macular neovascularization in eyes with large drusen. *Ophthalmology*, 127, 637–647.

Piccolino, F. C., Rigault de la Longrais, R., Ravera, G., Eandi, C. M., Ventre, L., Abdollahi, A., et al. (2005). The foveal photoreceptor layer and visual acuity loss in central serous chorioretinopathy. *American Journal of Ophthalmology*, 139, 87–99.

Ranjan, R., Agarwal, M., & Verma, N. (2020). Microrip of retinal pigment epithelium in central serous chorioretinopathy. *JAMA Ophthalmology*, 138, e193120.

Sato, T., Kishi, S., Watanabe, G., Matsumoto, H., & Mukai, R. (2007). Tomographic features of branching vascular networks in polypoidal choroidal vasculopathy. *Retina*, 27, 589–594.

Shinojima, A., Kawamura, A., Mori, R., Fujita, K., & Yuzawa, M. (2016). Findings of optical coherence tomographic angiography at the choriocapillaris level in central serous chorioretinopathy. *Ophthalmologica*, 236, 108–113.

Song, I. S., Shin, Y. U., & Lee, B. R. (2012). Time-periodic characteristics in the morphology of idiopathic central serous chorioretinopathy evaluated by volume scan using spectral-domain optical coherence tomography. *American Journal of Ophthalmology*, 154, 366–375.e4.

Wang, M., Munch, I. M., Hasler, P. W., Prünte, C., & Larsen, M. (2008). Central serous chorioretinopathy. *Acta Ophthalmologica*, 86, 126–145.

Yang, L., Jonas, J. B., & Wei, W. (2013). Optical coherence tomography-assisted enhanced depth imaging of central serous chorioretinopathy. *Investigative Ophthalmology & Visual Science*, 54, 4659–4665. F.

Yap, E. Y., & Robertson, D. M. (1996). The long-term outcome of central serous chorioretinopathy. *Archives of Ophthalmology*, 114, 689–692.

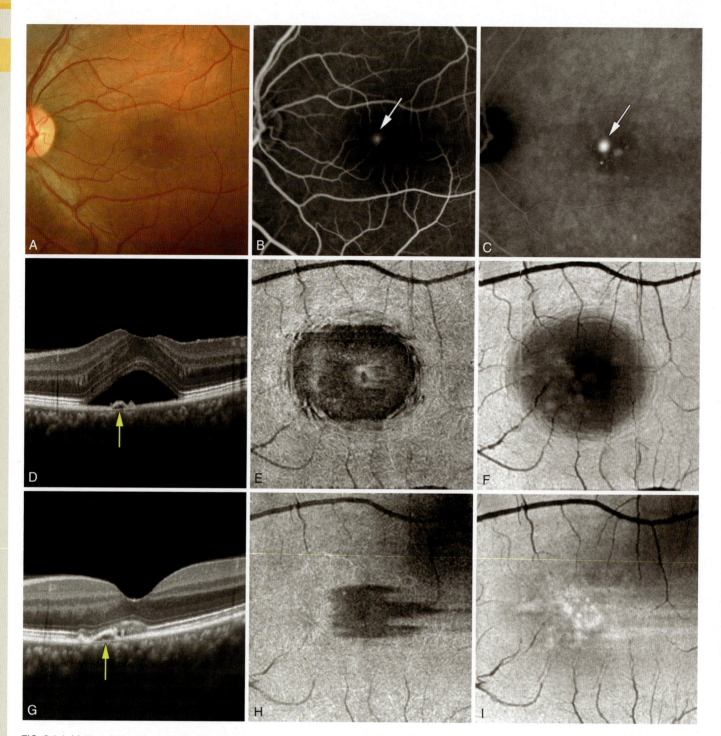

FIG. 8.1.1 Multimodal imaging of a patient with acute central serous chorioretinopathy. (A) Fundus photography shows a fovea neurosensory retinal detachment. (B) Fluorescein angiography and (C) indocyanine green angiography indicate an "inkblot" leakage *(white arrows)*. (D) Baseline OCT B-scan shows a serous detachment of the neurosensory retina and a serous pigment epithelium detachment (PED) *(yellow arrow)*. Baseline structural en face OCT segmented at the inner plexiform membrane (IPL) (E), and retinal pigment epithelium (RPE) (F) shows a circular hyporeflective area corresponding to signal loss secondary to subretinal fluid blockage. (G) Follow-up OCT B-scan shows subretinal fluid regressions with the serous PED's persistence *(yellow arrow)*. Follow-up en face OCT segmented at the level of IPL (H) and RPE (I) shows regression of the hyporeflective area.

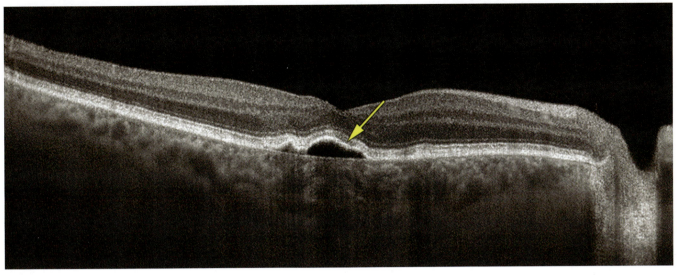

FIG. 8.1.2 OCT B-scan of a patient with central serous chorioretinopathy, associated with serous pigmented epithelium detachment *(yellow arrow)*.

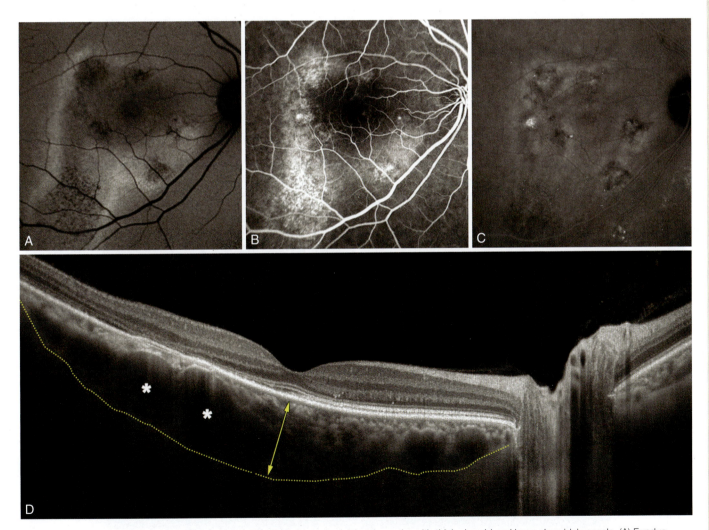

FIG. 8.1.3 Multimodal imaging of a patient with inactive central serous chorioretinopathy with thick choroid and large choroidal vessels. (A) Fundus autofluorescence was able to identify the classic descending tract sign associated with areas of hyperautofluorescence and hypoautofluorescence. (B) Fluorescein angiography shows areas of hyperfluorescence due to retinal pigment epithelium defect. (C) Indocyanine green angiography shows areas of hyperpermeability. (D) On the OCT B-scan, it is possible to identify a thickened choroid *(yellow dotted line and yellow arrow)* and dilated choroidal vessels *(white asterisks)*.

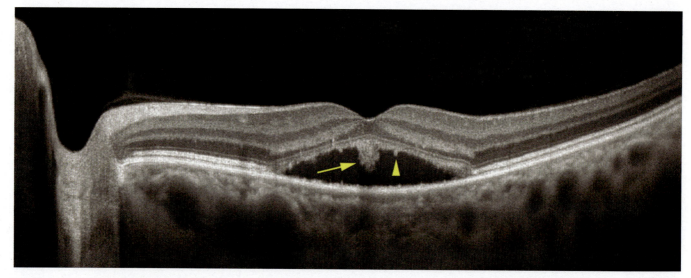

FIG. 8.1.4 OCT B-scan of a patient with acute central serous chorioretinopathy, associated with granulated changes of the outer photoreceptors layers *(yellow arrow and arrowhead)*.

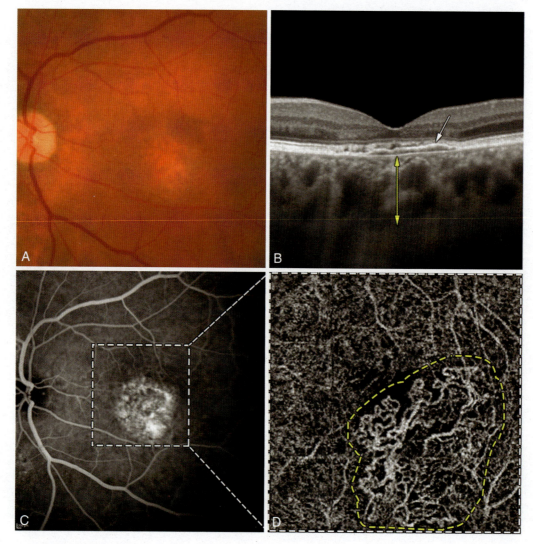

FIG. 8.1.5 Multimodal imaging of a patient with chronic central serous chorioretinopathy with secondary choroidal neovascularization. (A) Fundus photography shows mottled retinal pigment epithelium (RPE) without the presence of intraretinal or subretinal hemorrhage. (B) OCT B-scan centered on the fovea shows a flat RPE detachment *(white arrow)* associated with little subretinal fluid and thickened choroid and large dilated vessel *(yellow arrow)*. (C) Midphase fluorescein angiography shows no noticeable leakage. (D) OCT angiogram segmented at the choriocapillaris indicates the neovascular membrane complex *(yellow dashed line)*.

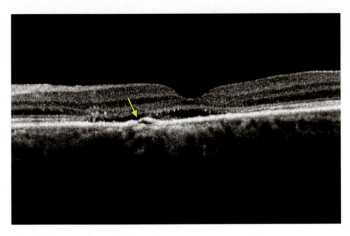

FIG. 8.1.6 OCT B-scan of a patient with chronic central serous chorioretinopathy, associated with retinal pigment epithelium microrip *(yellow arrow)*.

Myopic Choroidal Neovascular Membrane

Darin R. Goldman

9.1

75

Summary

Myopic choroidal neovascular membrane (CNV) is the most common non–age-related macular degeneration (AMD) cause for CNV. High myopia results in degenerative changes to Bruch's membrane and the retinal pigment epithelium (RPE) underlying the macula, which results in CNV formation in more than 10% of highly myopic eyes (Grossniklaus & Green, 1992). The associated exudation, hemorrhage, and/or scarring contribute to associated visual impairment. Although the natural history of myopic CNV tends to be more favorable than that of CNV secondary to AMD, without treatment, a significant portion of eyes will lose vision. Therefore, myopic CNV is a major cause for serious vision loss and blindness worldwide. With the rising prevalence of high myopia, this is likely to become an increasingly encountered macular condition. Anti–vascular endothelial growth factor (anti-VEGF) therapy has emerged as the most effective treatment for myopic CNV, although its use remains off-label in most countries. The OCT appearance of myopic CNV is often more subtle than that seen in other causes of CNV and sometimes can be overlooked if this is the only modality relied on for diagnosis (Figs. 9.1.1 and 9.1.2).

Key OCT Features

- Myopic CNV appears as a highly reflective, well-circumscribed, round complex on OCT.
- Typically, minimal associated exudation such as cystoid macular edema or subretinal fluid is present.
- Additional diagnostic modalities, such as fluorescein angiography, are often required to confirm the diagnosis of myopic CNV (Figs. 9.1.3 and 9.1.4).

REFERENCE

Grossniklaus, H. E., & Green, W. R. (1992). Pathologic findings in pathologic myopia. *Retina, 12*(2), 127–133.

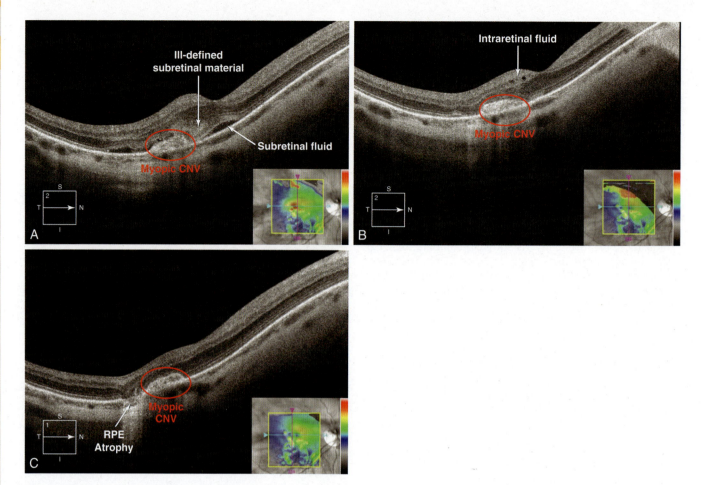

FIG. 9.1.1 (A) Myopic CNV appears as a somewhat ill-defined hyperreflective, dome-shaped elevation in the subretinal space between the neurosensory retina and the RPE. Associated subretinal fluid and less well-defined subretinal material with mixed reflectivity are present. (B) At 1 month after initial anti-VEGF therapy, the CNV complex becomes better defined, and the associated exudation is mostly resolved with some residual intraretinal fluid. (C) At 2 months after monthly anti-VEGF therapy, all associated fluid has resolved. The CNV has regressed into an area of subretinal fibrosis, and a small area of RPE atrophy has appeared. *CNV,* Choroidal neovascular membrane; *RPE,* retinal pigment epithelium; *VEGF,* vascular endothelial growth factor. (Modified with permission from Goldman, D. (In press). Choroidal neovascularization, not AMD. In: J. Duker & M. Liang M (Eds.), *Anti-VEGF use in ophthalmology*.)

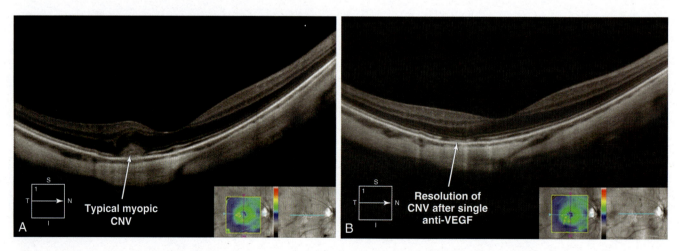

FIG. 9.1.2 (A) Typical myopic CNV identified as a dome-shaped hyperreflective elevation between the neurosensory retina and retinal pigment epithelium. There is no associated exudation. (B) After treatment with a single anti-VEGF injection, the CNV complex completely resolved. *CNV,* Choroidal neovascular membrane; *VEGF,* vascular endothelial growth factor.

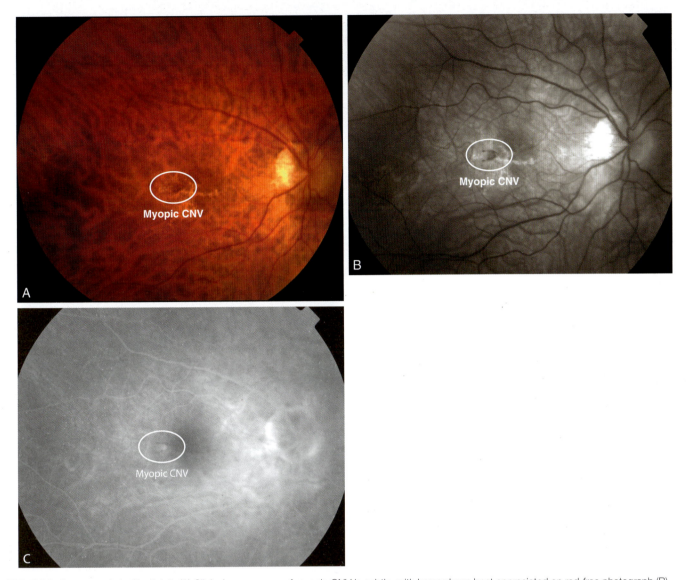

FIG. 9.1.3 Corresponds to Fig. 9.1.2. (A) Clinical appearance of myopic CNV is subtle, with hemorrhage best appreciated on red-free photograph (B). (C) Fluorescein angiography reveals a type 2 leakage pattern. *CNV*, Choroidal neovascular membrane.

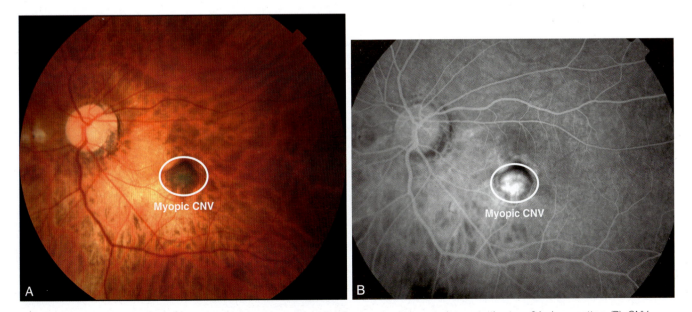

FIG. 9.1.4 (A) Typical myopic CNV clinical appearance and corresponding fluorescein angiogram demonstrating type 2 leakage pattern (B). *CNV*, Choroidal neovascular membrane

Myopic Macular Schisis

Darin R. Goldman

9.2

Summary

Myopia is one of the most common causes for macular schisis. Other causes include juvenile X-linked retinoschisis, optic pits, and idiopathic. Macular schisis in the setting of high myopia is thought to be due to a mechanical effect as a result of abnormal axial elongation and progressive sclera thinning. Subsequent stretching or splitting of the macular layers occurs due to the induced abnormal vitreoretinal tractional forces. A more descriptive term, "myopic ectatic retinopathy," representative of this presumed mechanism, has been proposed (Tsilimbaris et al., 2016). The schisis plane commonly occurs between the outer plexiform layer (OPL) and Henle fiber layer (HFL). However, the plane may occur in the inner, middle, or outer macular layers. No OCT-based epidemiologic studies have investigated the incidence and prevalence of myopic macular schisis. Myopic macular schisis appears to be more common with increasing degree of myopia/axial length and in the setting of posterior staphyloma. Visual acuity may be variably affected, and over time, myopic macular schisis is slowly progressive. Treatment is considered when visual symptoms or acuity progressively worsen. Interventions include vitrectomy with or without internal limiting membrane peeling and/or gas tamponade.

Key OCT Features

- Schisis may occur in multiple layers of the macula; however, the outer layers are most commonly affected, leaving a thicker inner retina and thinner outer retina.
- Perpendicular strands stretching within the schisis cavity are thought to be Müller cells.
- Other associated features of myopia may be noted on OCT, such as staphyloma, RPE atrophy, and vitreomacular interface abnormalities (Figs. 9.2.1–9.2.6).

REFERENCE

Tsilimbaris, M. K., Vavvas, D. G., & Bechrakis, N. E. (2016). Myopic foveoschisis: An ectatic retinopathy, not a schisis. *Eye (London), 30*(2), 328–329.

BIBLIOGRAPHY

Gohil, R., Sivaprasad, S., Han, L. T., Mathew, R., Kiousis, G., & Yang, Y. (2015). Myopic foveoschisis: A clinical review. *Eye (London), 29*(5), 593–601.

Ober, M. D., Freund, K. B., Shah, M., Ahmed, S., Mahmoud, T. H., Aaber, T. M., et al. (2014). Stellate nonhereditary idiopathic foveomacular retinoschisis. *Ophthalmology, 121*(7), 1406–1413.

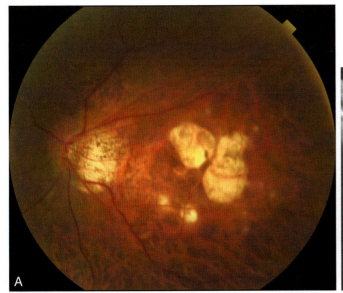
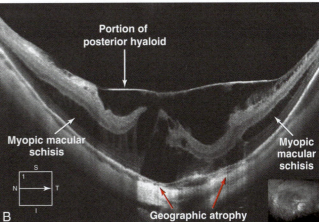

FIG. 9.2.1 (A) Fundus photograph of typical myopic macular schisis with significant atrophic myopic degeneration. (B) Corresponding OCT shows typical myopic macular schisis with a plane of separation located within the outer retinal layers.

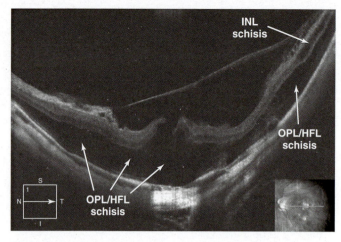

FIG. 9.2.2 Myopic macular schisis located within the OPL/HFL. A small affected area of schisis is seen within the INL. *HFL*, Henle fiber layer; *INL*, inner nuclear layer; *OPL*, outer plexiform layer.

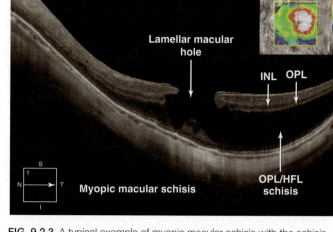

FIG. 9.2.3 A typical example of myopic macular schisis with the schisis plane located between the OPL and HFL. The INL is identified to help with orientation. A lamellar macular hole is present, which is commonly associated with myopic macular schisis. *HFL*, Henle fiber layer; *INL*, inner nuclear layer; *OPL*, outer plexiform layer.

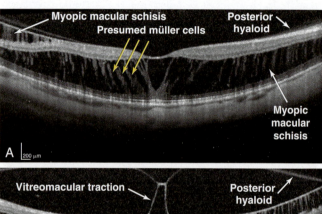

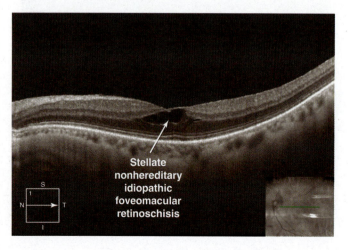

FIG. 9.2.5 An additional example of myopic macular schisis affecting the outer retinal layers.

FIG. 9.2.4 The right eye (A) and left eye (B) show features similar to those of myopic macular schisis in multiple layers. The posterior hyaloid is still adherent to the macula in the right eye but is lifting off in the left eye with associated vitreomacular traction. A tractional element may be contributing to the schisis in this case, along with the pathologic anatomic changes associated with myopia.

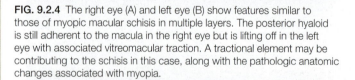

FIG. 9.2.6 Stellate nonhereditary idiopathic foveomacular retinoschisis is an entity with an OCT appearance similar to that of myopic macular schisis. However, the affected patient has neither myopia nor any known hereditary predisposing risk factors.

Dome-Shaped Macula

Darin R. Goldman

Summary

A dome-shaped macula describes an inward or convex indentation beneath the macula that is distinct from posterior staphyloma and evident only on OCT imaging. They occur in approximately 20% of highly myopic eyes. Although the pathogenesis is not clearly understood, the best theory surmises that variation in scleral thickness under the macula results in a localized region where a dome-shaped, relative, inward bulge occurs (Imamura et al., 2011). There is often an associated "cap" of subretinal fluid (hyporeflective space) in the absence of concomitant choroidal neovascular membrane (CNV). This fluid may be associated with larger domes and decreased visual acuity, is unresponsive to treatment, is typically nonprogressive, and is of unknown pathogenesis. The macular convexity associated with dome-shaped macula is most commonly oriented horizontally (Liang et al., 2015) and therefore is best visualized on a vertically oriented OCT B-scan (Fig. 9.3.1). Dome-shaped macula is more likely to occur in younger patients with longer axial lengths.

Key OCT Features

- There is inward bowing of the sclera within the central macula; the overlying macula follows the same contour, giving it an arched structure.
- A vertically oriented OCT scanning plane is most likely to detect the presence of a dome-shaped macula, although it may also be evident on a horizontally oriented OCT scan (Fig. 9.3.2).
- When a hyporeflective subretinal cavity/cap is present, this usually does not signify the presence of CNV.

REFERENCES

Imamura, Y., Iida, T., Maruko, I., Zweifel, S. A., & Spaide, R. F. (2011). Enhanced depth imaging optical coherence tomography of the sclera in dome-shaped macula. *American Journal of Ophthalmology*, *151*(2), 297–302.

Liang, I. C., Shimada, N., Tanaka, Y., Nagaoka, N., Moriyama, M., Yoshida, K., et al. (2015). Comparison of clinical features in highly myopic eyes with and without a dome-shaped macula. *Ophthalmology*, *122*(8), 1591–1600.

BIBLIOGRAPHY

Caillaux, V., Gaucher, D., Gualino, V., Massin, P., Tadayoni, R., & Gaudric, A. (2013). Morphologic characterization of dome shaped macula in myopic eyes with serous macular detachment. *American Journal of Ophthalmology*, *156*(5), 958–967.

Gaucher, D., Erginay, A., Lecleire-Collet, A., Haouchine, B., Ruech, M., Cohen, S. -Y., et al. (2008). Dome-shaped macula in eyes with myopic posterior staphyloma. *American Journal of Ophthalmology*, *145*(5), 909–914.

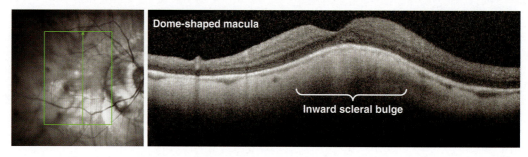

FIG. 9.3.1 Vertically oriented OCT scan reveals an inward bulge of the scleral in the central macula, which is typical of dome-shaped macula.

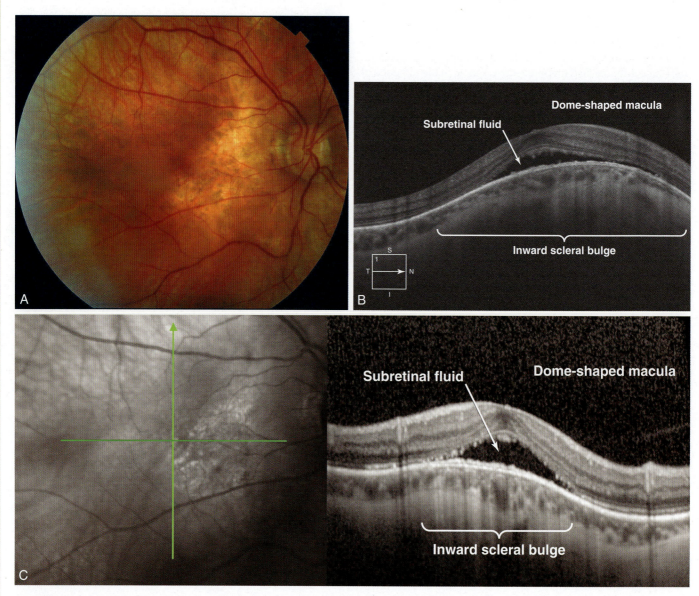

FIG. 9.3.2 (A) Color photograph in a high myope with a posterior staphyloma. (B) Horizontally oriented OCT scan reveals a dome-shaped macula with corresponding inward bulging of the underlying sclera. Subretinal fluid is present, which did not change over a prolonged period with and without treatment. (C) Vertically oriented OCT scan reveals the same features as in part B; however, the dome-shaped elevation is less obvious, which is atypical.

Posterior Staphyloma

Darin R. Goldman

9.4

Summary

Axial elongation occurs as the globe enlarges in pathologic myopia. Along with this elongation, localized outward protrusions in the globe wall termed "posterior staphyloma" can occur. These areas have a steeper curvature than the surrounding globe wall. Many types of posterior staphyloma have been described (Hsiang et al., 2008), the most common being ovoid shaped and involving the central macula and optic nerve (Frisina et al., 2016). The presence of posterior staphyloma is strongly correlated with the degree of myopia and is present in as many as 50% of eyes with pathologic myopia (Ohno-Matsui et al., 2017). Detection of posterior staphyloma on a purely clinical basis can be difficult in milder cases. The depth-resolved nature of OCT image acquisition makes this imaging modality particularly useful for detecting staphyloma, especially those in a peripapillary or macular location (Fig. 9.4.1 and 9.4.2). Additional macular pathologic conditions are commonly found in concert with staphyloma, such as schisis, choroidal neovascular membrane (CNV), epiretinal membrane, vitreomacular traction (VMT), and tractional detachment. Identification of staphyloma should raise suspicion for identifying these additional entities.

Key OCT Features

- The normal horizontal appearance of retinal layers on OCT is lost in posterior staphyloma, giving way to a posterior bowing.
- Posterior bowing of the retina, choroid, and sclera occurs at the edges of a staphyloma.
- OCT is most useful to identify both peripapillary and macular staphyloma.
- Identification of macular staphyloma should raise suspicion for other concomitant macular pathologic processes associated with high myopia (Fig. 9.4.3).

REFERENCES

Hsiang, H. W., Ohno-Matsui, K., Shimada, N., Hayashi, K., Moriyama, M., Yoshida, T., et al. (2008). Clinical characteristics of posterior staphyloma in eyes with pathologic myopia. *American Journal of Ophthalmology, 146*(1), 102–110.

Frisina, R., Baldi, A., Semeraro, F., Cesana, B. M., & Parolini, B. (2016). Morphological and clinical characteristics of myopic posterior staphyloma in Caucasians. *Graefes Arch Clin Exp Ophthalmol, 254*(11) 2199–2129.

Ohno-Matsui, K., Alkabes, M., Salinas, C., Mateo, C., Moriyama, M., Cao, K., et al. (2017). Features of posterior staphylomas analyzed in wide-field fundus images in patients with unilateral and bilateral pathological myopia. *Retina, 37*(3), 477–486.

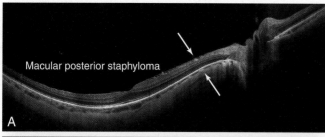

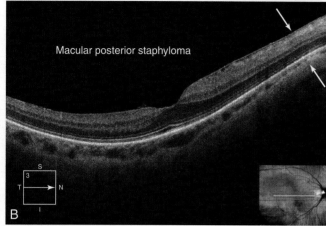

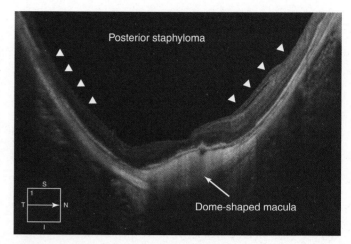

FIG. 9.4.1 (A) Wide-angle OCT view of macular posterior staphyloma. There is a point of deflection adjacent to the optic nerve where the sclera bows outward along with the overlying retina and choroid (between *arrows*). The staphyloma is present temporal to this point and extends off the area imaged. (B) Higher magnification OCT view of same macular staphyloma.

FIG. 9.4.2 Posterior staphyloma involving the posterior pole encompassing the optic nerve (not pictured) and macula. There is a high radius of curvature at the edges of the macula *(arrowheads)*. Note that a dome-shaped macula is also present (see Chapter 9.3), which accounts for the relatively flatter foveal contour. (With permission from Duker, J. W., Waheed, N. K., & Goldman, D.R. (2014). *Handbook of retinal OCT: Optical coherence tomography* (9.1, pp. 46–47). Philadelphia: Saunders.)

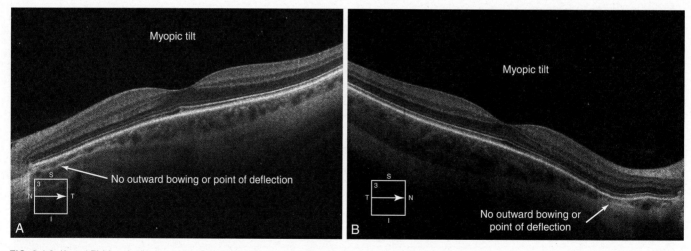

FIG. 9.4.3 (A and B) Myopic tilt should be distinguished from posterior staphyloma. Myopic tilt is common with lower degrees of myopia. There is a generalized diagonal sloping of the macula. However, distinct from posterior staphyloma, there is no outward bowing or point of deflection.

Hydroxychloroquine Toxicity | 10.1

Carlos A. Moreira Neto | Joao Victor Peres Lima

Summary

Several systemic medications can cause retinal toxicity. One group of these drugs is antimalarial. Chloroquine use can cause retinal toxicity in 10% of patients, whereas hydroxychloroquine causes retinal toxicity in 3% of patients (Marmor et al., 2016; Melles & Marmor, 2014). These rates are dose dependent and time dependent and also depend on other systemic conditions, such as impaired renal function and concomitant use of tamoxifen. Rates of toxicity increase when the dose is greater than 5 mg/kg/day of body weight and when the drug is used for greater than 5 years (Tsang et al., 2015).

The disease presents with fundus, fluorescein, OCT, and visual field changes (Marmor et al., 2016). Early stages of toxicity can stop progressing with drug withdrawal, while severe advanced toxicity with damage to the RPE can progress even after drug suspension (Marmor et al., 2016; Tsang et al., 2015).

OCT changes in their possible order of appearance are as follows:

Parafoveal disruption of the integrity of the myoid/ellipsoid/photoreceptor zone (Fig. 10.1.1):

- Earlier stage of involvement, with preserved central subfoveal area.
- Loss of outer cone segments and architectural disruption, most evident inferior and temporal (Cukras et al., 2015).
- These changes are often asymptomatic and stop progressing with drug withdrawal.
- Diffuse external retinal involvement and photoreceptors distress (Fig. 10.1.2):

- The subfoveal region may show hypertransmission signal.
- The bull's eye maculopathy aspect appears only in advanced stages with irreversible visual damage (Sisternes et al., 2015).
- Diffuse loss of photoreceptors and external disorganization (Fig. 10.1.3):
- Inner retina maintains its architecture and thickness is preserved.
- Collapse of foveal depression associated with evident disorganization of the external retina (loss of the outer retinal layers—inner segments [IS]/outer segments [OS]/ellipsoid zone [EZ]) (Marmor et al., 2016; Tsang et al., 2015).

REFERENCES

Cukras, C., Huynh, N., Vitale, S., Wong, W. T., Ferris, F. L., & Sieving, P. A. (2015). Subjective and objective screening tests for hydroxychloroquine toxicity. *Ophthalmology, 256*, 1807–2816..

Marmor, M. F., Kellner, U., Lai, T. Y. Y., Melles, R. B., Mieler, W. F., & the American Academy of Ophthalmology, (2016). Recommendations on screening for chloroquine and hydroxychloroquine retinopathy. *Ophthalmology, 123*(6), 1386–1394.

Melles, R. B., & Marmor, M. F. (2014). The risk of toxic retinopathy in patients on long-term hydroxychloroquine therapy. *JAMA Ophthalmology, 132*(12), 1453–1460.

Sisternes, L., Hu, J. L., Rubin, D. L., & Marmor, M. F. (2015). Localization of damage in progressive hydroxychloroquine retinopathy on and off the drug: Inner versus outer retina, parafovea versus peripheral fovea. *Investigative Ophthalmology & Visual Science, 56*, 3415–3426.

Tsang, A. C., Ahmadi, P. S., Virgili, G., Gottlieb, C. C., Hamilton, J., & Coupland, S. G. (2015). Hydroxychloroquine and chloroquine retinopathy: A systematic review evaluating the multifocal electroretinogram as a screening test. *Ophthalmology, 122*, 1239–1251.

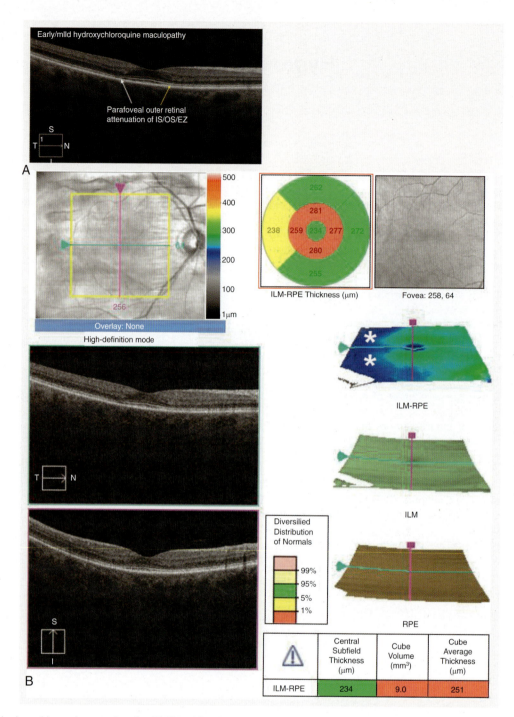

FIG. 10.1.1 Early hydroxychloroquine maculopathy. (A) Signs of early maculopathy are more evident temporally (*white arrow*) than nasally (yellow arrow). Temporally, there is attenuation of the inner segments/outer segments/ellipsoid zone. (B) Corresponding OCT thickness map illustrating mild thinning of the outer retina in a parafoveal distribution *(asterisks and red box). ILM,* Inner limiting membrane; *RPE,* retinal pigment epithelium.

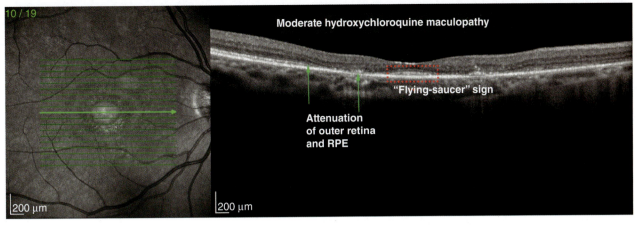

FIG. 10.1.2 Moderate hydroxychloroquine maculopathy. Outer retinal loss *(between green arrows)*. Disruption of inner segments/outer segments/ellipsoid zone, with preserved inner retina and no evident signals of hypertransmission in the subfoveal area, represented by the "flying saucer" sign (red dotted rectangle). *RPE*, retinal pigment epithelium.

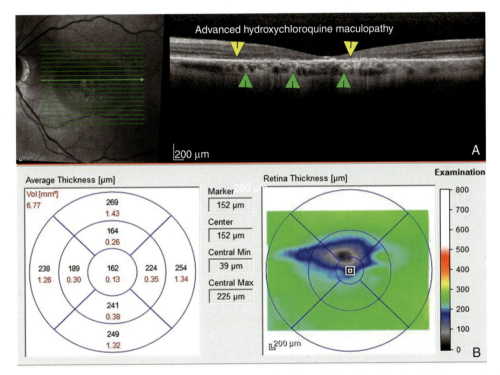

FIG. 10.1.3 Advanced hydroxychloroquine maculopathy. (A) Diffuse external involvement and disruption of outer retina layers and retinal pigment epithelium (RPE) *(between yellow arrowheads)*. Localized reverse shadowing *(green arrowheads)* is identified due to a significant RPE dropout. (B) Thickness map shows a profound macular atrophy.

Pentosan Toxicity

Shilpa J. Desai

10.2

Summary

Pentosan polysulfate sodium is a drug used to treat symptoms of interstitial cystitis (bladder pain, urinary frequency, and urgency). This drug has been approved for use since 1996, but only in 2018 was the connection made between chronic exposure to the drug and toxicity to the retinal pigment epithelium (RPE) (Pearce et al., 2018). Since that time, multiple studies have demonstrated a dose-response relationship to pentosan exposure and retinal toxicity. Imaging findings of this toxicity include hyperpigmented spots in the fovea, yellow deposits, and patchy RPE loss (Fig. 10.2.1) (Hanif et al., 2019). Fundus autofluorescence reveals densely packed hypoautofluorescence and hyperautofluorescence in the macula, along with RPE atrophy (Fig. 10.2.2). Finally, OCT shows RPE loss and nodular deposits (Fig. 10.2.3). The macular RPE loss results in decreased central acuity. The exact pathophysiology of this toxicity is not well understood. The only known prevention is to avoid using medication (Vora et al., 2020).

Key Features

- Pentosan polysulfate sodium is a drug used to treat interstitial cystitis with a dose-dependent retinal toxicity.
- Pentosan toxicity is associated with RPE loss and atrophy resulting in loss of vision.
- The most classic finding is densely packed speckled autofluorescence in the macula.

REFERENCES

Hanif, A. M., Shah, R., Yan, J., Varghese, J. S., Patel, S. A., Cribbs, B. E., et al. (2019). Strength of association between pentosan polysulfate and a novel maculopathy. *Ophthalmology*, *126*(10), 1464–1466.

Pearce, W. A., Chen, R., & Jain, N. (2018). Pigmentary maculopathy associated with chronic exposure to pentosan polysulfate sodium. *Ophthalmology*, *125*(11), 1793–1802.

Vora, R. A., Patel, A. P., & Melles, R. (2020). Prevalence of maculopathy associated with long-term pentosan polysulfate therapy. *Ophthalmology*, *127*(6), 835–836.

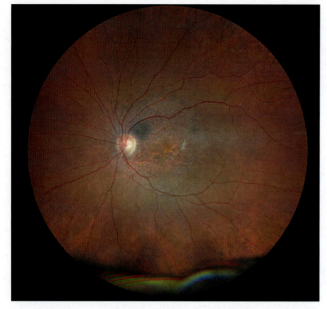

FIG. 10.2.1 Fundus photo in pentosan toxicity shows areas of hyperpigmentation, yellow deposits, and spots of atrophy. (Courtesy of Shilpa J. Desai.)

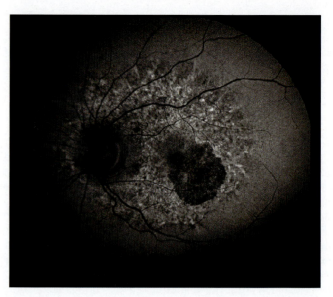

FIG. 10.2.2 Fundus autofluorescence of pentosan toxicity shows classic densely packed hypofluorescence and hyperfluorescence.

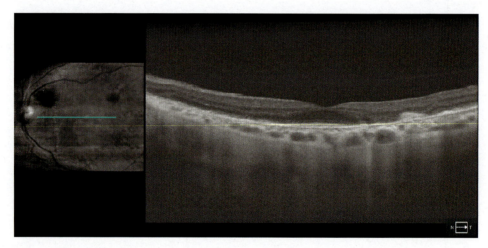

FIG. 10.2.3 OCT in pentosan toxicity shows areas of atrophy and subretinal deposits.

Vitelliform Dystrophy

Shilpa J. Desai | A. Yasin Alibhai

11.1

Summary

Vitelliform dystrophy is defined as an abnormal accumulation of lipofuscin in or under the retinal pigment epithelium (RPE) layer of the retina (Agrawal, 2012). Vitelliform dystrophy is typically inherited in an autosomal dominant pattern and thought to be caused by a defect in the peripherin/retinal degeneration slow (RDS) gene (Schatz et al., 2003).

Onset is typically between 30 and 50 years of age. Patients may report a decrease in vision or metamorphopsia. The vision loss in vitelliform dystrophy is typically mild, with many patients diagnosed during a screening eye examination while asymptomatic.

Retinal examination will show a yellow or pigmented deposit in the macula. The disease is typically bilateral, but may be asymmetric. Fluorescein angiography will show blockage at the area of lipofuscin deposition with late hyperfluorescence of the lesion resulting from staining (Fig. 11.1.1). OCT will show deposits in or beneath the RPE layer (Fig. 11.1.2). Vitelliform dystrophy can be associated with subretinal fluid or choroidal neovascularization (CNV).

The differential diagnosis of vitelliform dystrophy includes other pattern dystrophies, including Best disease, age-related macular degeneration, choroiditis, and idiopathic CNV.

Treatment of vitelliform dystrophy is typically monitoring unless CNV occurs. In that case, anti–vascular endothelial growth factor agents are indicated.

Key Features

- Vitelliform dystrophy is an abnormal accumulation of lipofuscin in the RPE layer of the retina.
- OCT shows deposits above the RPE.
- Over time, regression of the deposits can occur and appear as hyporeflective lucency underlying the retina.
- Vitelliform dystrophy can be associated with subretinal fluid or CNV.
- Treatment is typically monitoring or treatment of associated CNV, if indicated.

REFERENCES

Agrawal, A. (2012). Heredodystrophic disorders affecting the pigment epithelium and retina. In: S. Desai (Ed.), *Gass' atlas of macular diseases* (5th ed., pp. 239–426). Philadelphia: Elsevier.

Schatz, P., Abrahamson, M., Eksandh, L., Ponjavic, V., Andréasson, S. (2003). Macular appearance by means of OCT and electrophysiology in members of two families with different mutations in RDS (the peripherin/RDS gene). *Acta Ophthalmologica Scandinavica*, 81(5), 500–507.

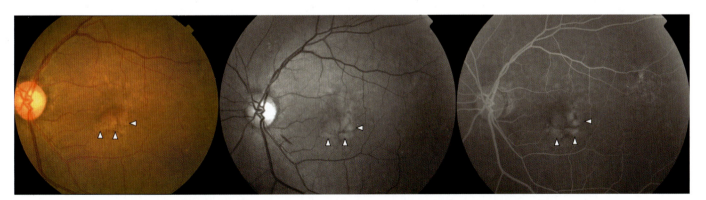

FIG. 11.1.1 Color fundus, red-free, and fluorescein angiography images showing accumulation of lipofuscin material at the fovea.

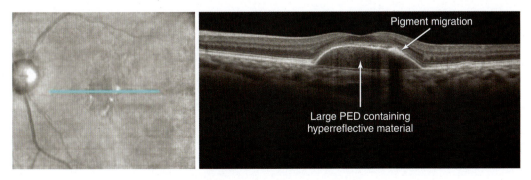

FIG. 11.1.2 OCT scan corresponding to Fig. 11.1.1. There is a large retinal pigment epithelium detachment with hyperreflective material within it, corresponding to the vitelliform lesion. *PED*, Pigment epithelial detachment.

Macular Telangiectasia

Carlos A. Moreira Neto

12.1

Summary

Macular telangiectasia (MacTel) manifests as retinal vascular anomalies in middle-aged or older adults. Abnormalities of the retinal capillary bed include vessel dilatation and tortuosity, aneurysms, vascular leakage, and deposition of hard exudates. Type I MacTel, thought to be a form of Coats' disease, is typically unilateral and is more commonly seen in males. Telangiectatic blood vessels are seen temporal to the macula and are associated with exudates. Type II MacTel is a bilateral disease with no sex predilection. There is a loss of the parafoveal retinal transparency with ectasia of temporal capillaries. Exudation is rarely seen in type II. With disease progression, crystal deposition and retinal pigment epithelium (RPE) hyperplasia can occur and choroidal neovascularization (CNV) may develop.

Key Points

Type I

- Male and unilateral.
- Presence of exudation (Fig. 12.1.1).
- OCT: Cystoid macular edema is most prominent feature, although subretinal fluid may be present (Fig. 12.1.2).

Type II

- Bilateral.
- Microaneurysmal abnormalities in the temporal parafovea (Fig. 12.1.3).
- RPE hyperplasia is present (Fig. 12.1.3).
- OCT: Area of low intraretinal reflectivity with lamellar defects at multiple layers typically located just temporal to the foveal center (Fig. 12.1.4).
- Pigment deposition and atrophy may develop with chronic disease.
- OCTA: Foveal avascular zone may become irregular, capillary drop out with reduced vascular density, distortion, and dragging (Fig. 12.1.5).

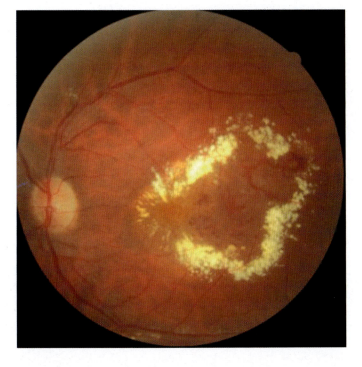

FIG. 12.1.1 Color fundus photograph shows macular exudation in a patient with type I macular telangiectasia.

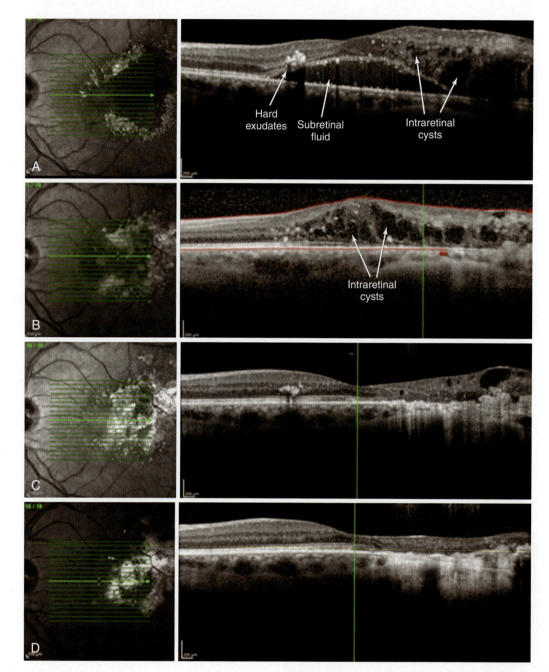

FIG. 12.1.2 OCT (corresponding to the eye with type I MacTel seen in Fig. 12.1.1) before (A) and after (B, C, D) treatment. (A) Note subretinal fluid and intraretinal cystic cavities of low and medium reflectivity and hyperreflective deposits within the retina, corresponding to hard exudates. Visual acuity 20/200. (B) OCT 3 months after treatment with focal grid laser and one intravitreal bevacizumab injection. Visual acuity 20/60. (C) OCT 3 months after second focal grid laser and one intravitreal bevacizumab injection. Visual acuity 20/30. (D) OCT 3 months after (C). Visual acuity 20/30.

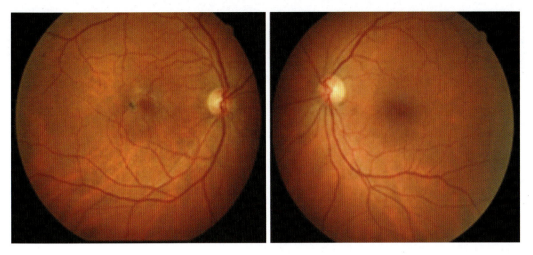

FIG. 12.1.3 Color fundus photos of a subject with type 2 MacTel show loss of the foveal reflex with subtle microaneurysmal abnormalities in the temporal parafoveal region in both eyes. Color photograph of the right eye also shows RPE clumping and hyperplasia along with foveal atrophy.

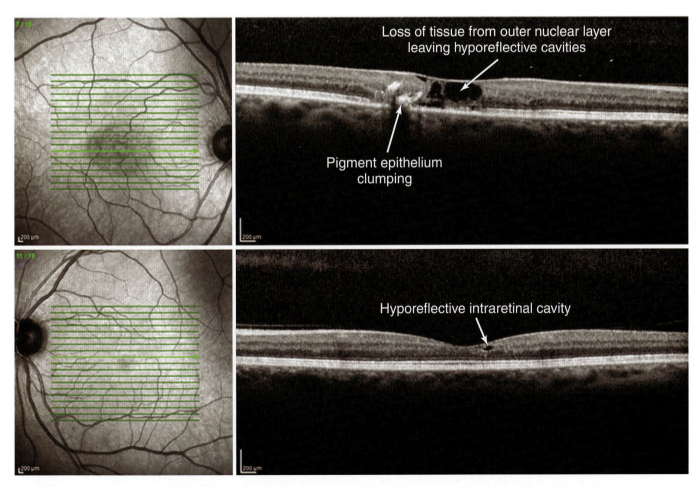

FIG. 12.1.4 OCT (corresponding to the subject in Fig. 12.1.3) in MacTel type 2. In the right eye *(top image)*, there is loss of tissue from outer nuclear layer and atrophy of inner segment/outer segment junction. In the left eye *(bottom image)*, there is an intraretinal hyporeflective cyst.

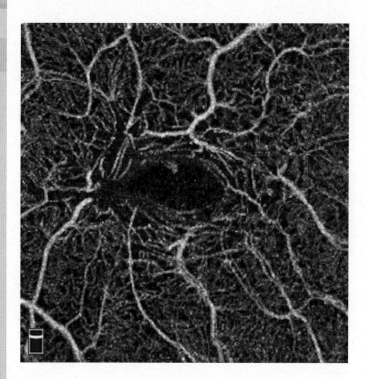

FIG. 12.1.5 OCT angiography shows superficial segmentation (corresponding to the right eye of the subject Fig. 12.1.3) in MacTel type 2. Note the irregular foveal avascular zone.

Isolated Cystoid Macular Edema | 13.1

Shilpa J. Desai | A. Yasin Alibhai

Summary

Cystoid macular edema (CME) is defined as retinal thickening in the macula due to leakage and accumulation of fluid in the intracellular spaces of the macula. Symptoms of CME include vision loss, decreased color/contrast sensitivity, metamorphopsia, micropsia, or scotoma. CME can be caused by a myriad of etiologies, most typically occurring following ocular surgery. Intraretinal fluid accumulates preferentially within the outer plexiform layer. Underlying photoreceptor function is affected by the fluid and changed architecture, which results in vision loss (Fig. 13.1.1). The clinical appearance is that of many small cystic cavities bunched together with the fovea into a petaloid arrangement (Fig. 13.1.2). Fluorescein angiography shows petaloid leakage in the macula. OCT shows cystic accumulation of fluid in the macula (Fig. 13.1.3). CME is most often self-limited. When treatment is required, it is geared toward the specific underlying cause, typically including topical and intravitreal corticosteroids (Fig.13.1.4).

Key Points

- CME is defined as retinal thickening within the macula.
- OCT shows large, hyporeflective cystic spaces located predominantly within the outer plexiform layer, although the inner plexiform and nuclear layers may also be involved.
- Severe cases may include spillover of fluid into the subretinal space.

BIBLIOGRAPHY

Afshar, A. R., Fernandes, J. K., Patel, R. D., Ksiazek, S. M., Sheth, V. S., Reder, A. T., et al. (2013). Cystoid macular edema associated with fingolimod use of multiple sclerosis. *JAMA Ophthalmology*, 113(1), 103–107.

Augustin, A., Loewenstein, A., & Kuppermann, B. D. (2010). Macular edema. General pathophysiology. *Developments in Ophthalmology*, 47, 10–26.

Rotsos, T. G., & Moschos, M. M. (2008). Cystoid macular edema. *Clinical Ophthalmology*, 24, 919–930.

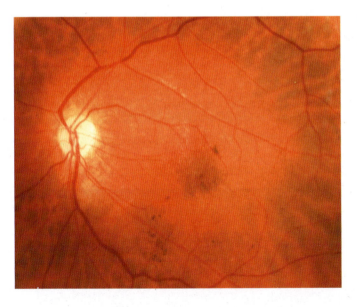

FIG. 13.1.1 Color fundus photograph showing loss of the normal foveal reflex due to cystoid macular edema in a patient status post vitrectomy for retinal detachment repair.

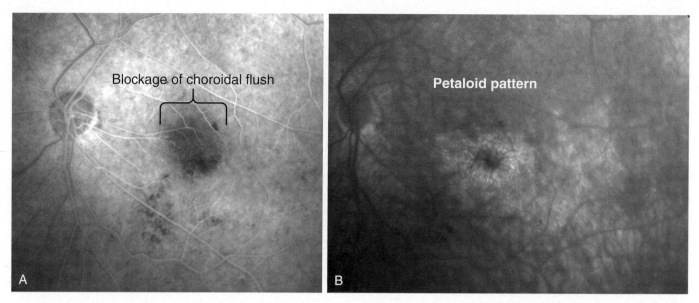

FIG. 13.1.2 Fluorescein angiogram corresponding to Fig. 13.1.1. Early phase (A) demonstrates blockage of choroidal flush from edema. Late phase image (B) shows leakage in a petaloid pattern.

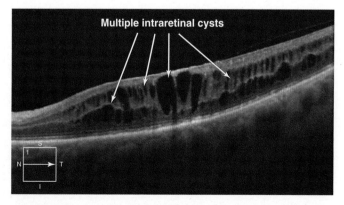

FIG. 13.1.3 OCT B-scan corresponding to Figs. 13.1.1 and 13.1.2. Retinal thickening and intraretinal fluid primarily in the outer plexiform layers are seen.

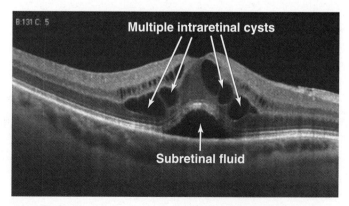

FIG. 13.1.4 OCT B-scan in a patient with pars planitis and severe cystoid macular edema shows multiple intra retinal cysts primarily in the outer plexiform layer, but also involving the inner nuclear layer. Additionally, subretinal fluid is present.

Angioid Streaks

Shilpa J. Desai | A. Yasin Alibhai

14.1

Summary

Angioid streaks are linear cracks in Bruch's membrane. They are caused by a breakdown in the collagen and elastic lamina of Bruch's membrane. There are a number of potential causes of angioid streaks, including pseudoxanthoma elasticum, Ehler-Danlos syndrome, Paget's disease, sickle cell disease, and other hemoglobinopathies (Paton, 1972). Angioid streaks may cause vision change in three different ways. First, the streak may travel through the fovea, leading to retinal pigment epithelium (RPE) loss. Mild trauma to the eye can cause rupture of the choroid, leading to submacular hemorrhage and vision loss. Finally, secondary choroidal neovascularization (CNV) can cause hemorrhage and macular edema. Clinical examination reveals orange-red to brown linear irregularities extending radially from the peripapillary region into the peripheral fundus. Fluorescein angiography shows irregular hyperfluorescence along the streak secondary to overlying RPE deposition (Fig. 14.1.1). OCT shows the angioid streaks in cross-section as a discontinuity in Bruch's membrane (Fig. 14.1.2). Although no specific treatment can address angioid streaks, any underlying systemic condition should be addressed. CNV is the main cause for vision loss and can be treated with anti–vascular endothelial growth factor therapy (Martinez-Serrano et al., 2016).

Key Points

- Angioid streaks are linear cracks in Bruch's membrane resulting from breakdown in the elastic and collagen lamina.
- Visual symptoms are caused by secondary hemorrhage or CNV.
- OCT shows breaks in the Bruch's membrane–RPE complex of an angioid streak in cross-section.
- Secondary CNV, which is type 2, can be effectively detected and monitored with OCT.

REFERENCES

Martinez-Serrano, M. G., Rodriguez-Reyes, A., Guerrero-Naranjo, J. L., Salcedo-Villanueva, G., Fromow-Guerra, J., García-Aguirre, G., et al. (2016). Long-term follow-up of patients with choroidal neovascularization due to angioid streak. *Clinical Ophthalmology, 11,* 23–30.

Paton, D. (1972). *The relation of angioid streaks to systemic disease.* Springfield, IL: Charles C Thomas.

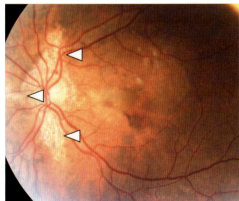 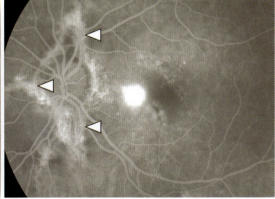

FIG. 14.1.1 Color fundus and fluorescein angiogram photographs show retinal pigment epithelium loss over angioid streaks radiating from the peripapillary zone *(white arrows)*. There is secondary CNV present within the nasal macula. *CNV,* Choroidal neovascularization.

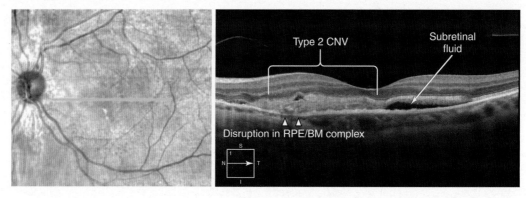

FIG. 14.1.2 OCT B-scan corresponding to Fig. 14.1.1. There are focal breaks in the RPE-BM complex in the area of an angioid streak. Subretinal fluid and subretinal hyperreflective material associated with a type 2 CNV lesion are also identified. *BM,* Bruch's membrane; *CNV,* choroidal neovascularization; *RPE,* retinal pigment epithelium.

X-Linked Juvenile Retinoschisis

Kate V. Hughes | Shilpa J. Desai*

Summary

X-linked retinoschisis or juvenile retinoschisis (XLJR) is an inherited disorder affecting only males. It is caused by mutations in the retinoschisin gene (*RS-1*). There is considerable variability in the onset and severity of the disease.

The clinical hallmarks are cystic retinal changes in the macula (stellate maculopathy) and peripheral retinal elevations as the result of retinoschisis (Figs. 14.2.1 and 14.2.2). Vitreous veils over the peripheral schisis, vitreous hemorrhage, and retinal detachment also can occur. OCT is the most useful imaging modality available to confirm the diagnosis.

Key OCT Features

- Splitting (schisis) of both inner and outer retinal layers occurs (Figs. 14.2.1 and 14.2.3).
- Posterior pole retinal cystic changes in both inner and outer retinal layers resemble cystoid macular edema but extend beyond the macula and do not result in extensive macular thickening.

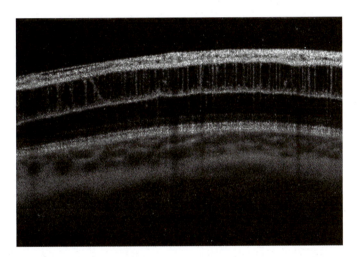

FIG. 14.2.1 X-linked schisis with OCT. Note splitting of both inner and outer retina with no evidence of retinal detachment.

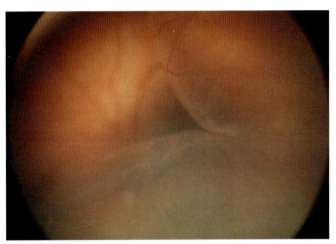

FIG. 14.2.2 Corresponding color fundus photograph showing extensive peripheral retina elevation from retinoschisis.

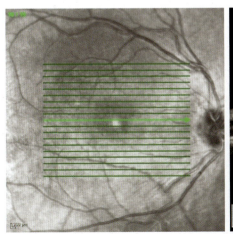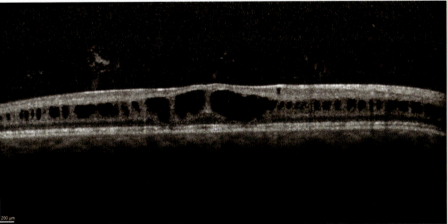

FIG. 14.2.3 Macular OCT of a 16-year-old male patient showing typical inner and outer schisis diffusely through the posterior pole.

*With contributions from Jay S. Duker

Phoebe L. Mellen | Shilpa J. Desai*

Summary

Ocular albinism can occur clinically in several forms. If only the eyes are involved, it is termed "ocular albinism," which is most frequently inherited as X-linked recessive (Grønskov et al., 2007). If both the skin and the eyes are affected, it is referred to as oculocutaneous albinism (OCA). OCA is most often inherited autosomal recessively. Clinically, the fundus is always hypopigmented, but it can be difficult in a young child to differentiate normal from disease (Kruijt et al., 2018). However, most affected children have nystagmus and iris transillumination defects (Fig. 14.3.1). Interestingly, affected individuals do not have nyctalopia or color vision problems. The classic clinical finding is blunting of the foveal light reflex (Fig. 14.3.2) (Kruijt et al., 2018). In patients with OCA, it is important to rule out Hermansky-Pudlak syndrome and Chediak-Higashi syndrome because these disorders can be associated with important hematologic abnormalities.

Key OCT Finding

- Absence or severe blunting of the foveal depression is present (Kruijt et al., 2018) (Fig. 14.3.3).
- OCTA shows persistence of the superficial capillary plexus and lack of a foveal avascular zone (FAZ) in some cases (Mansour et al., 2021).

REFERENCES

Grønskov, K., Ek, J., & Brondum-Nielsen, K. (2007). Oculocutaneous albinism. *Orphanet Journal of Rare Diseases 2*, 43.

Kruijt, C. C., de Wit, G. C., Bergen, A. A., Florijn, R. A., Schalij-Delfos, N. E., & van Genderen, M. M. (2018). The phenotypic spectrum of albinism. *Ophthalmology*, *125*, 1953–1960.

Mansour, H. A., Uwaydat, S., Yunis, M. H., & Mansour, A. M. (2021). Foveal avascular zone in oculocutaneous albinism. *BMJ Case Reports*, *14*, e240208.

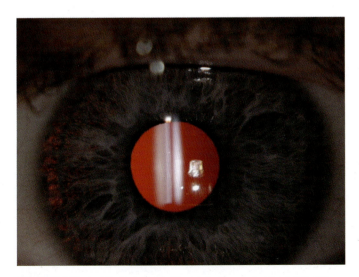

FIG. 14.3.1 Typical iris transillumination defects are visualized with retro-illumination.

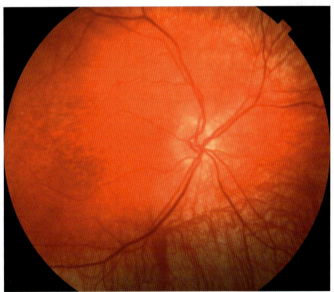

FIG. 14.3.2 Representative fundus photograph of a patient with oculocutaneous albinism. There is blunting of the foveal reflex and hypopigmentation of the entire fundus.

*With contributions from Jay S. Duker

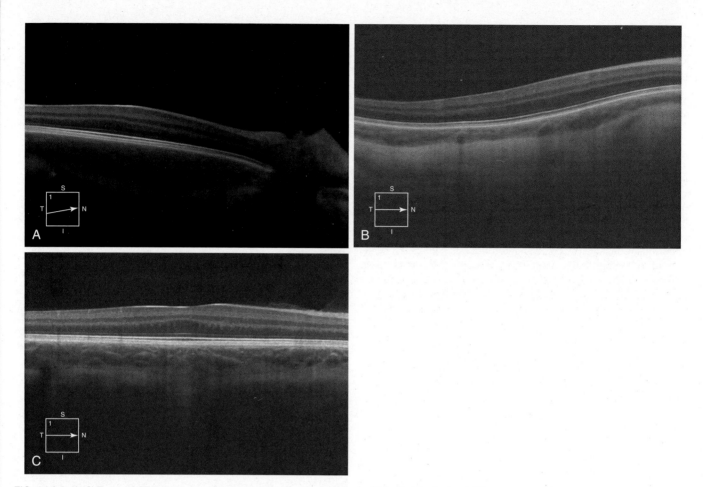

FIG. 14.3.3 (A–C) Typical OCT appearance of albinism in three different patients. Note that the horizontal B-scans were obtained such that the central fovea was bisected in all patients. However, the foveal hypoplasia with retention of the inner retinal layers is the key feature of disease.

Subretinal Perfluorocarbon

14.4

Phoebe L. Mellen | Shilpa J. Desai*

Summary

Perfluorocarbon (PFC) is a dense, synthetic liquid used during vitrectomy surgery to flatten the retina. Inadvertent migration of this liquid into the potential subretinal space is possible. OCT is the most definitive diagnostic modality for detecting the presence of subretinal PFC, with which it has a distinct appearance. It is important to differentiate this entity from other subretinal pathologic conditions in which management can be entirely different (Lesnoni et al., 2004).

Key OCT Features

- There is a dome-shaped, hyporeflective space with a round top and flat bottom, located under the retina (Figs. 14.4.1 and 14.4.2).
- The internal reflectivity is comparable to the normal vitreous cavity.
- The overlying retinal layers are bunched into a thin sheet and appear mostly hyperreflective.
- Reverse shadowing, with hyperreflective retinal pigment epithelium (RPE) and choroid, may be present beneath the bubble.

REFERENCE

Lesnoni, G., Rossi, T., & Gelso, A. (2004). Subfoveal liquid perfluorocarbon. *Retina*, *24*, 172–176.

---

*With contributions from Jay S. Duker

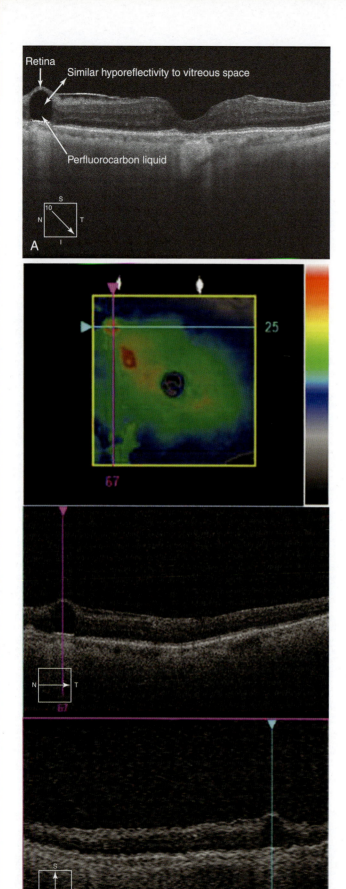

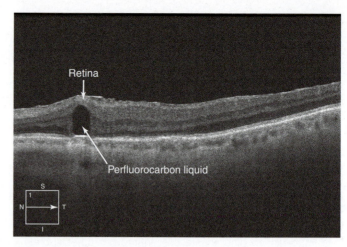

FIG. 14.4.2 Perfluorocarbon liquid bubble underneath the macula showing characteristic features, including round top, flat bottom, and compressed overlying retina.

FIG. 14.4.1 (A) Structural OCT shows perfluorocarbon (PFC) liquid underneath the nasal macula. (B) Thickness map is shown, centered on PFC bubble.

Diabetic Macular Edema   15.1
Nadia K. Waheed

Summary

Diabetic macular edema (DME) is characterized by thickening and edema of the macula that can develop at any stage of diabetic retinopathy. High blood glucose levels damage the retinal microcirculation, resulting in abnormal permeability and ischemia. Increased vessel permeability results in fluid and lipid-rich exudate leakage into the surrounding retina, distorting normal retinal architecture, and reduces visual acuity if near the fovea (Figs. 15.1.1 and 15.1.2). Clinically significant macular edema has been largely replaced by macular edema involving the center as an indication for treatment in the era of anti–vascular endothelial growth factor. OCT is the most important ancillary test in DME diagnosis, monitoring treatment, and following progression. OCTA may show the features characteristic of the stage of diabetic retinopathy as described in the appropriate diabetic retinopathy chapters

Key OCT Features

- Subretinal fluid accumulation and intraretinal fluid accumulation are the key features of DME that are evident on OCT (Fig. 15.1.3).
- There is decreased reflectivity of outer retinal layers on OCT due to increased foveal thickness.
- Exudates can be seen as hyperreflective spots within the retina.

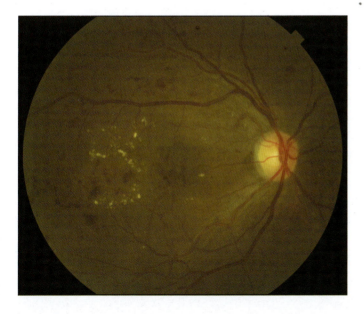

FIG. 15.1.1 Color fundus image shows hard exudates, intraretinal hemorrhages, microaneurysms, and cotton wool spots.

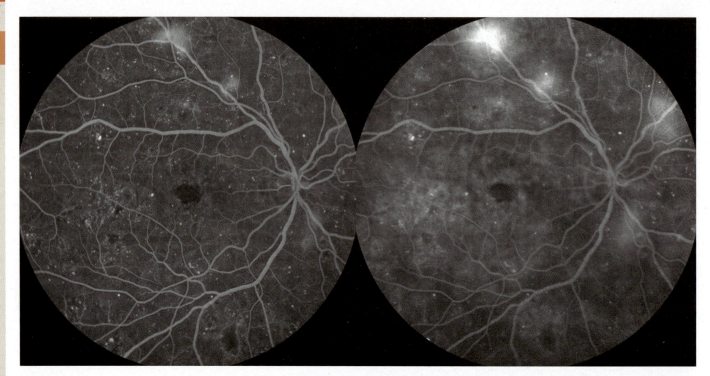

FIG. 15.1.2 Early frame fluorescein angiography highlights the microaneurysms, and late phase shows diffuse leakage across the posterior pole of the retina.

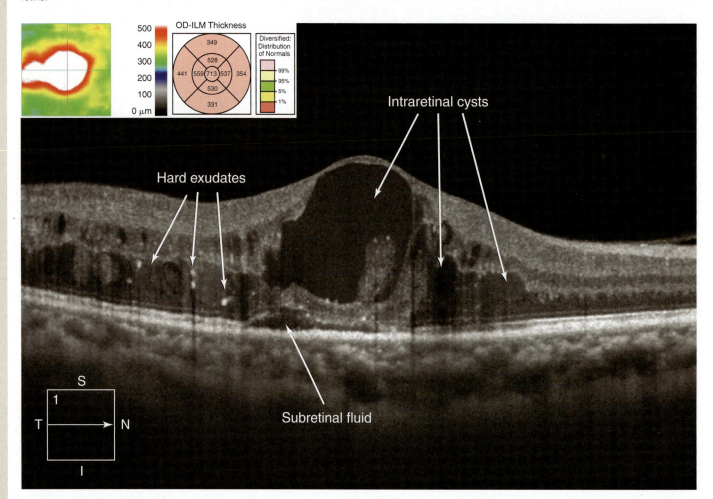

FIG. 15.1.3 OCT B-scan through the central macula shows thickening with cystic changes. The area and extent of thickening can be visualized by the false color rendering of the thickness map over the C-scan *(inset)*. The retinal thickness map also provides quantitative information about thickening. Hard exudates can be seen as a hyperreflective cluster. There is also a trace of subretinal fluid with overlying distortion of the inner segment/outer segment/ellipsoid zone. *ILM*, Inner limiting membrane.

Summary

Nonproliferative diabetic retinopathy (NPDR) represents the earliest stages of retinopathy caused by diabetes. Damage to the small blood vessels of the retina can result in the formation of nerve fiber layer infarcts (cotton wool spots), hard exudates (Fig. 15.2.1), and intraretinal hemorrhages. Other microvascular abnormalities, including microaneurysms and dilated or tortuous vessels, also can develop (Fig. 15.2.2). Venous beading and intraretinal microvascular abnormalities (IRMAs) can arise in severe NPDR. NPDR is classified into mild, moderate, and severe based on the risk for developing neovascularization. Vision loss in NPDR primarily occurs from the development of diabetic macular edema (DME), which can occur at any stage of the disease (Fig. 15.2.3). OCTA may show microaneurysms, perifoveal capillary remodeling with enlargement of the foveal avascular zone (FAZ) and eventually macular ischemia. Widefield OCTA may show areas of capillary dropout and resulting ischemia (Fig 15.2.4).

Key OCT Features

- Hard exudates appear as hyperreflective clusters in the retina.
- Microaneurysms (MAs) have homogeneous inner reflectivity and an outer rim of hyperreflectivity.
- Cotton wool spots manifest as areas of hyperreflectivity within the nerve fiber layer.
- OCT angiography (OCTA) may show microaneurysms, capillary remodeling, and capillary dropout.

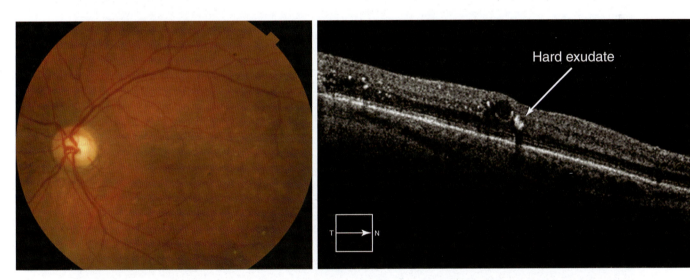

FIG. 15.2.1 Color fundus image and corresponding OCT scan shows hard exudate. Hard exudates appear as irregularly shaped, intraretinal, hyperreflective lesions on OCT imaging.

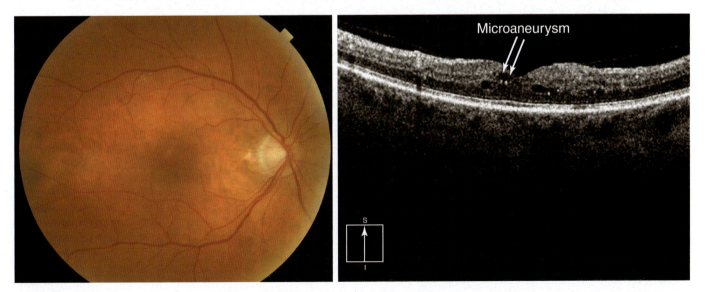

FIG. 15.2.2 Color fundus image and corresponding OCT scan show microaneurysms.

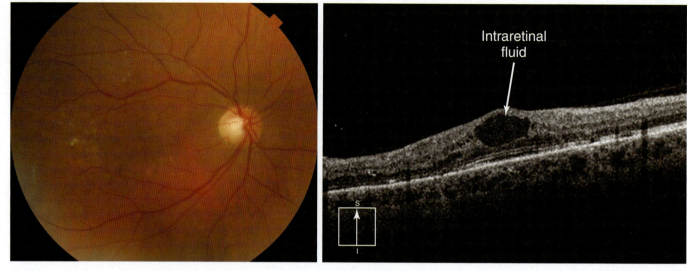

FIG. 15.2.3 Color fundus image and corresponding OCT scan show intraretinal fluid.

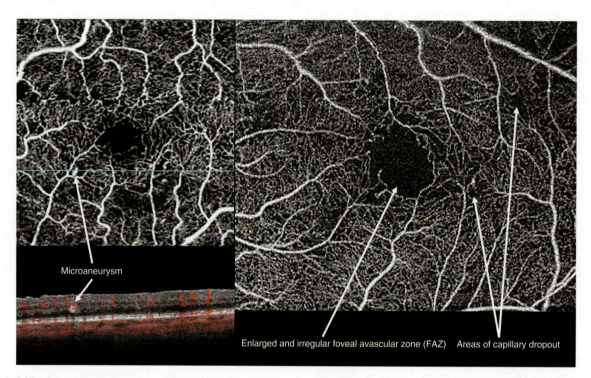

FIG. 15.2.4 OCTA shows microaneurysms, capillary remodeling around the FAZ and capillary dropout.

Proliferative Diabetic Retinopathy | 15.3

Nadia K. Waheed | Antonio Yaghy

Summary

High blood glucose levels over a prolonged period damage the retinal microvasculature and result in ischemia. In response, factors such as vascular endothelial growth factor are released from ischemic retina, inducing the formation of new blood vessels. These new blood vessels are often fragile and prone to leaking. Proliferative diabetic retinopathy (PDR) is characterized by neovascularization arising from the optic disc and retina, which may cause preretinal and vitreous hemorrhage (Figs. 15.3.1 and 15.3.2). Subsequent fibrosis of the new vessels creates tractional forces leading to retinal detachment (Fig. 15.3.3). Vision loss may occur as a result of PDR-induced hemorrhage, but this often resolves as a result of reabsorption of blood. Vision loss because of macula-involved tractional detachment is generally permanent. OCT is quite useful in documenting the presence of tractional retinal detachments within the macula, particularly if the area affected is shallowly detached. OCTA shows all the characteristic features of NPDR, along with more severe ischemia. Neovascular fronds can be seen protruding into the vitreous and these can be observed to regress after therapy (Fig. 15.3.4).

Key Points

- PDR is characterized by the formation of new retinal blood vessels.
- Neovascularization on OCT can be seen as loops of hyper-reflective blood vessels protruding into the retina.
- Tractional retinal detachments are defined by the presence of subretinal fluid. They are distinguished by overlying tractional bands.

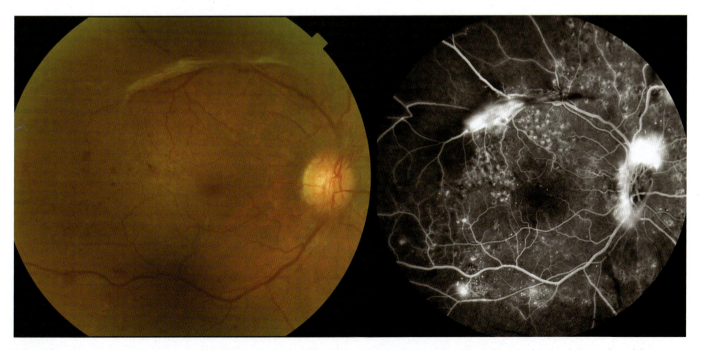

FIG. 15.3.1 Neovascularization of the superior temporal arcade of the retina and optic disc is seen on both the color fundus photograph and the accompanying fluorescein angiogram.

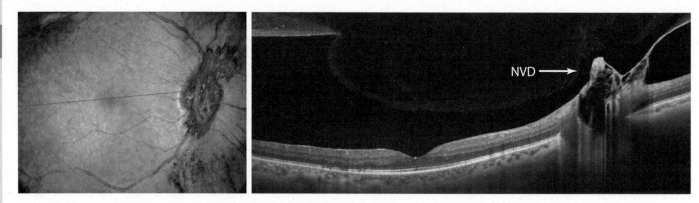

FIG. 15.3.2 OCT scan corresponding to Fig. 15.3.1. Line scan through the area of the neovascularization of the optic disc reveals hyperreflective neovascularization into the vitreous cavity. *NVD,* Neovascularization of the disc.

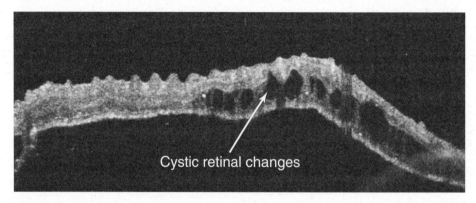

FIG. 15.3.3 Tractional retinal detachment seen on OCT corresponds to superotemporal neovascularization seen in Fig. 15.3.1. There is thickening of the retina with associated cystic changes.

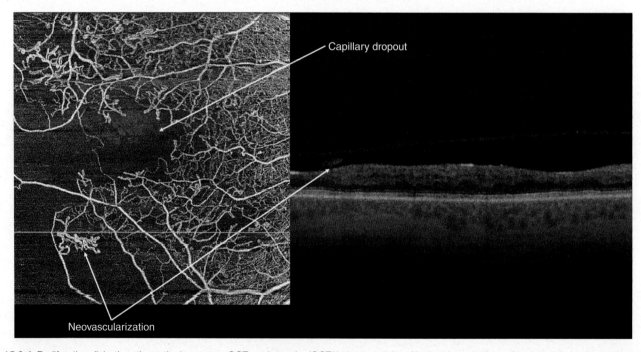

Fig 15.3.4 Proliferative diabetic retinopathy images on OCT angiography (OCTA) show peripheral ischemia and areas of neovascularization seen on the OCTA and confirmed by the position of the neovascularization protruding through the internal limiting membrane on cross-sectional scans with flow overlay *(right).*

Branch Retinal Vein Occlusion

16.1

Caroline R. Baumal | Angell Shi

Summary

Branch retinal vein occlusion (BRVO) is caused by occlusion of one of the branches of the central retinal vein. The pathogenesis is related to mechanical compression from an atherosclerotic tributary of the retinal artery, degenerative vascular changes, and thrombus formation. Hypercoagulability may play a role in some cases. It is the second most common retinovascular disorder after diabetic retinopathy. The 5-year incidence is 0.6% and increases with age. The age of onset is variable, but typically between 60 to 70 years old. Risk factors include hypertension, cardiovascular disease, hyperlipidemia, obesity, and glaucoma. Diagnosis can usually be made with clinical examination alone, revealing dilation and tortuosity of the obstructed branch retinal vein associated with retinal hemorrhages. Cotton wool spots, lipid exudate, macular edema, retinal neovascularization, and capillary nonperfusion may be features (Fig. 16.1.1A). A sclerotic retinal vein may be the only sign of a prior retinal vein occlusion. Retinal imaging with OCT and fluorescein angiography can aid in prognostication and determination of therapy (Fig. 16.1.1.B–C). BRVO usually has a good prognosis (Fig. 16.1.2A–D). Visual acuity depends on the area of retinal ischemia and status of the fovea. Assessment and reduction of systemic risk factors are indicated to reduce the occurrence of another BRVO. Treatment of the sequelae of BRVO (specifically macular edema or neovascularization) may include anti–vascular endothelial growth factor (VEGF) agents, intraocular corticosteroids, and laser photocoagulation.

Key OCT Findings

- OCT is key to diagnose macular edema, determine if the fovea is involved, and follow response to therapy.
- OCT findings include cystoid macular edema, intraretinal hyperreflectivity from hemorrhages, shadowing from edema and hemorrhages, and subretinal fluid.
- After resolution of CME, disruption of the foveal photoreceptor layer, specifically the ellipsoid layer and external limiting membrane, has been associated with poorer visual prognosis.

BIBLIOGRAPHY

Kang, H. M., Chung, E. J., Kim, Y. M., & Koh, H. J. (2013). Spectral-domain optical coherence tomography (SD-OCT) patterns and response to intravitreal bevacizumab therapy in macular edema associated with branch retinal vein occlusion. *Graefe's Archive for Clinical and Experimental Ophthalmology 251*, 501–508.

Lim, H. B., Kim, M. S., Jo, Y. J., & Kim, J. Y. (2015). Prediction of retinal ischemia in branch retinal vein occlusion: Spectral-domain optical coherence tomography study. *Investigative Ophthalmology & Visual Science, 56*(11), 6622–6629.

Spaide, R. F., Lee, J. K., Klancnik, J. K., Jr., & Gross, N. E. (2003). Optical coherence tomography of branch retinal vein occlusion. *Retina 23*(3), 343–347.

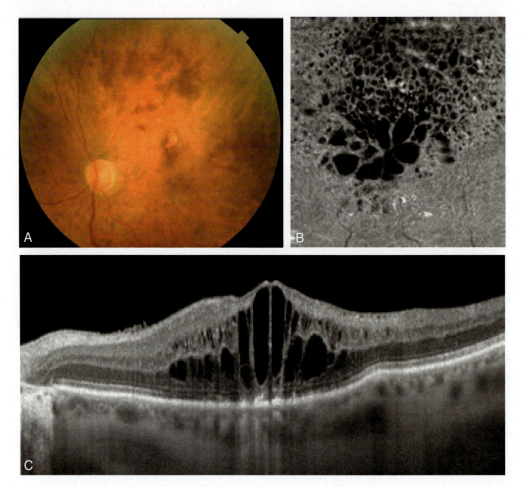

FIG. 16.1.1 (A) Color photo of a superotemporal branch retinal vein occlusion in a 75-year-old man presenting with a 3-month history of blurred vision (acuity 20/100). Note retinal hemorrhages following the superotemporal vein, as well as lipid exudate inferior to the fovea, cotton wool spots, and collateral vessels superior to the optic nerve. (B) En face image reveals large dark microcysts around the fovea and smaller cysts extending superiorly. (C) Spectral-domain OCT reveals intraretinal cysts, hyperreflective foci and disruption of the external limiting membrane, interdigitation zone, and ellipsoid zone in the center of the fovea.

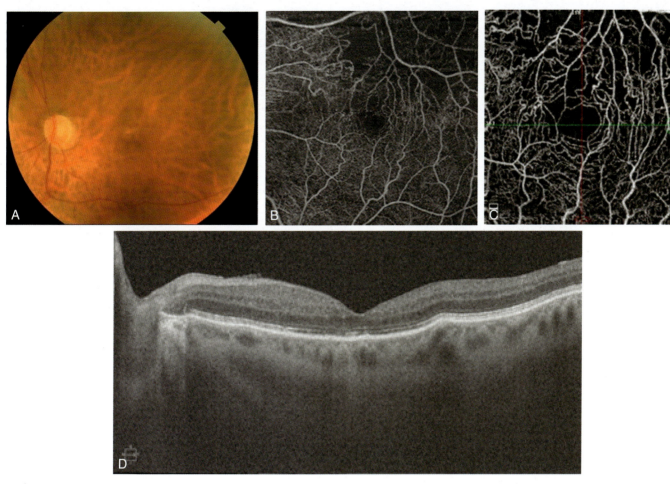

FIG. 16.1.2 (A) Color photo 1 year later after six anti–vascular endothelial growth factor injections with complete resolution of retinal hemorrhage, foveal granularity, sheathing of the superotemporal retinal veins, and collateral vessels superior to the optic nerve and temporal to the macula. Visual acuity measured 20/60. (B) 6 mm × 6 mm OCT angiography image (OCTA) demonstrates areas of capillary nonperfusion as well as collateral vessels superonasal to the fovea. (C) 3 mm × 3 mm OCTA of the same regions shows widened intercapillary spaces superior to the fovea, in contrast to the normal circulation below the fovea. (D) SD-OCT shows resolution of macular edema with some residual external limiting membrane and ellipsoid discontinuity.

Central Retinal Vein Occlusion | 16.2

Nadia K. Waheed | Caroline R. Baumal | Antonio Yaghy

Summary

Central retinal vein occlusion (CRVO) results from occlusion of the central retinal vein at or proximal to the lamina cribrosa. The central retinal vein is the major venous drainage system for the inner retina, and disruption of flow can result in severe visual loss from ischemia, macular edema, and/or neovascularization. The pathogenesis of CRVO is hypothesized to follow the principles of Virchow's triad for venous thrombosis, involving vascular wall damage, stasis of blood flow, and hypercoagulability. The prevalence and 15-year incidence of CRVO are 0.2%.

Risk factors include elderly age, diabetes mellitus, hyperlipidemia, hypertension, cardiovascular disease, obesity, ocular hypertension, glaucoma, and hypercoagulable states.

CRVO is classified as either nonischemic, which is a milder form, or as ischemic; this has implications for prognosis and treatment. Clinical findings include dilation and tortuosity of the retinal veins and retinal hemorrhages in all four quadrants (Fig. 16.2.1A–C), optic disc edema, cotton wool spots (nerve fiber layer infarcts), lipid exudate, cystoid macular edema, retinal ischemia, and later sequelae of iris and angle neovascularization leading to glaucoma in ischemic CRVO subtypes. Fluorescein angiography findings include delayed venous filling, retinal capillary nonperfusion, staining of retinal veins, retinal edema, and neovascularization. Treatment includes maximizing control of systemic risk factors, intravitreal injection of anti–vascular endothelial growth factor (anti-VEGF) or corticosteroid agents, and panretinal laser photocoagulation for significant neovascularization.

Key OCT Features

- OCT is key to diagnosing associated macular edema, evaluating the involved retinal layers, and determining response to therapy (Figs. 16.2.2 and 16.2.3).
- Visual acuity inversely correlates with macular thickening measured with OCT.
- After treatment of macular edema, discontinuity of the photoreceptors (especially the ellipsoid zone) and retinal architecture correlate with worse visual acuity.
- OCT angiography (OCTA) shows vessel dilation and tortuosity and associated macular edema (Fig 16.2.4).

BIBLIOGRAPHY

Laouri, M., Chen, E., Looman, M., & Gallagher, M. (2011). The burden of disease of retinal vein occlusion: Review of the literature. *Eye (London)*, *25*(8), 981–988.

Martinet, V., Guigui, B., Glacet-Bernard, A., Zourdani, A., Coscas, G., Soubrane, G., et al. (2012). Macular edema in central retinal vein occlusion: Correlation between optical coherence tomography, angiography and visual acuity. *International Ophthalmology*, *32*(4), 369–377.

Shin, H. J., Chung, H., & Kim, H. C. (2011). Association between integrity of foveal photoreceptor layer and visual outcome in retinal vein occlusion. *Acta Ophthalmologica*, *89*, e35–e40.

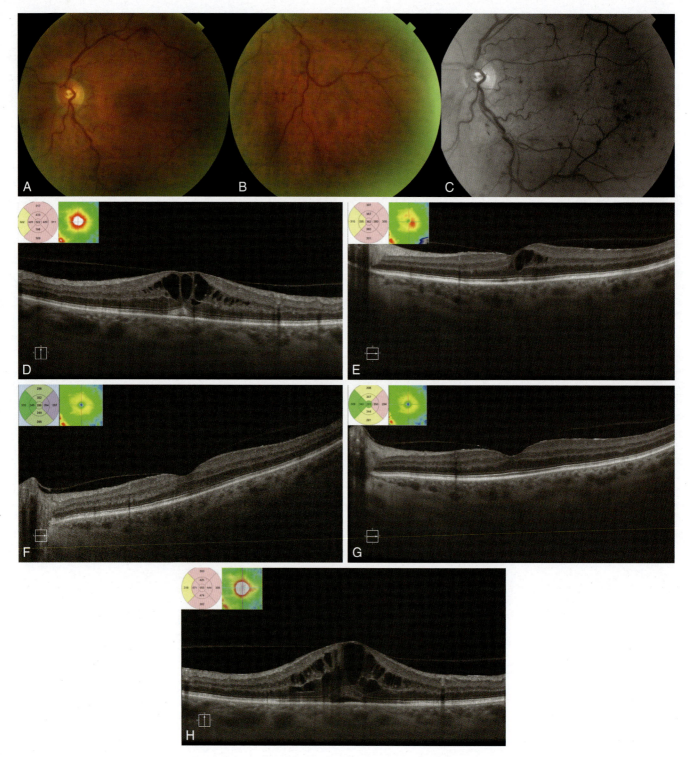

FIG. 16.2.1 (A–C) Color and red-free photographs of a patient presenting with mild central retinal vein occlusion and cystoid macular edema (CME). (D) OCT B-scan reveals CME with large central cysts in the inner nuclear layer and smaller perifoveal cysts. Note the vitreomacular attachment. First anti–vascular endothelial growth factor (VEGF) injection was given. (E) At 4 weeks after anti-VEGF treatment, the central subfoveal thickness is reduced to 362 and acuity improved to 20/40. (F) At 3 months after two anti-VEGF injections, cystoid macular edema resolved and acuity returned to 20/20. Anti-VEGF injection was given. (G) After three anti-VEGF injections, the CME was completely resolved. At this time no treatment was given. (H) CME recurred 6 months after presentation with a central subfoveal thickness of 655 microns. Her last anti-VEGF was 3 months before recurrence of CME.

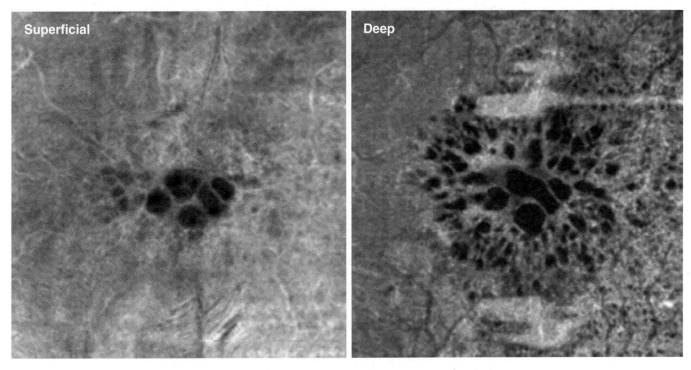

FIG. 16.2.2 En face images highlight that black cysts are more prominent in the deep retina than the superficial retina.

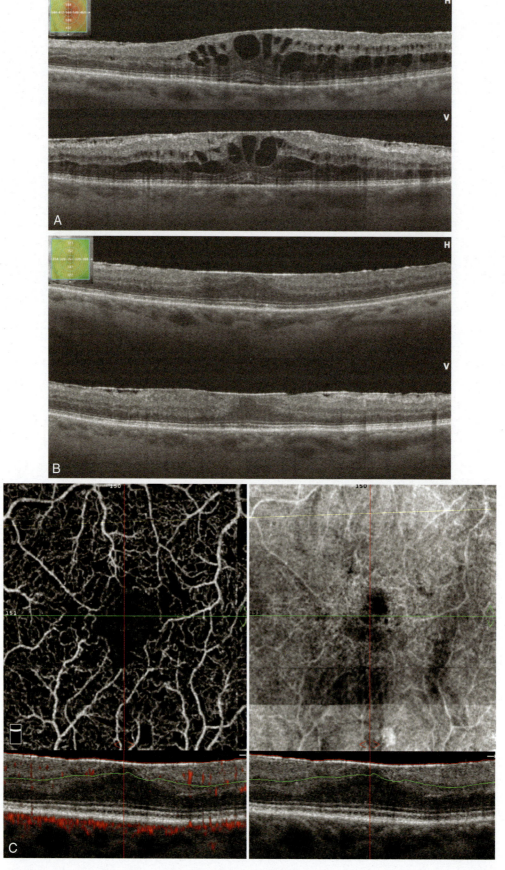

FIG. 16.2.3 (A) Two OCT B-scans centered on the fovea. Intraretinal cysts are large centrally and decrease in size in the perifoveal region. A small amount of subretinal fluid and an epiretinal membrane can be seen. Central foveal thickness measures 560 μm. (B) Four weeks after anti–vascular endothelial growth factor treatment, the cysts have resolved but the residual epiretinal membrane is apparent. (C) OCT angiography shows abnormally widened capillary spaces even though no CME is present.

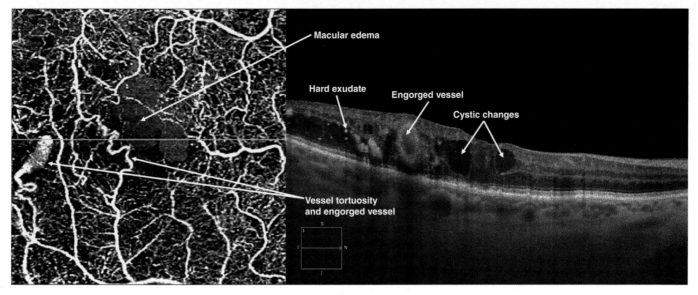

Fig 16.2.4 OCT angiography of central retinal vein occlusion shows vessel tortuosity, engorgement, and ischemia.

Branch Retinal Artery Occlusion

17.1

Caroline R. Baumal | Matthew N. Henderson

Summary

Branch retinal artery occlusion (BRAO) results from obstruction of one of the branches of the central retinal artery. The most common etiology is emboli secondary to either carotid plaques or cardiac disease, although other embolic sources have been reported. Less common, nonembolic causes include vasospasm and inflammatory and hypercoagulable disorders. Medical evaluation of cardiovascular and carotid disease is indicated due to the association with increased morbidity and mortality. Patients are typically 70 years or older and present with painless, unilateral, partial visual loss. Amaurosis fugax preceding persistent loss of vision may represent emboli, causing temporary occlusion of the retinal artery with subsequent released into the distal circulation. Location of the BRAO is often at the retinal artery bifurcation where the artery lumen is narrower. Ischemic retinal whitening and inner retinal edema develop along the path of the occluded branch artery. Other features include visible emboli in 60% of eyes, vessel attenuation and narrowing, segmentation of blood flow, known as boxcarring, and cotton-wool spots. Clinical features are usually diagnostic in acute BRAO, but fluorescein angiography (FA) and OCT are useful to demonstrate BRAO features (Fig. 17.1.1). OCT can assist in trending structural retinal changes and identify inner retinal atrophy and loss of the inner retinal layered architecture in eyes after acute BRAO findings have resolved.

Key OCT Findings

- OCT can demonstrate the structural damage to the inner retina in BRAO.
- Acutely, OCT demonstrates inner retinal layer hyperreflectivity and thickening due to ischemic swelling in the affected area.
- Inner retinal changes in acute BRAO can shadow details of the underlying outer retinal layers.
- Acute phase OCT findings may also include middle retinal layer hyperreflectivity and thickening at the level of the inner nuclear layer (INL), termed "paracentral acute middle maculopathy" (PAMM).
- In chronic BRAO, OCT reveals inner retinal and nerve fiber layer (NFL) atrophy with preservation of the outer nuclear layer (ONL) and adjacent photoreceptor/retinal pigment epithelium (RPE) layers.
- OCT angiography (OCTA) can characterize flow deficits in acute BRAO eyes to differentiate the involvement of the inner retinal plexuses.

BIBLIOGRAPHY

Bonini Filho, M.A., Adhi, M., de Carlo, T.E., Ferrara, D., Baumal, C.R., Witkin, A.J., et al. (2015). Optical coherence tomography angiography in retinal artery occlusion. *Retina 35*(11), 2339–2246. doi:10.1097/IAE.0000000000000850. PMID: 26457398.

Chen, X., Rahimy, E., Sergott, R. C., Nunes, R. P., Souza, E. C., Choudhry, N., et al. (2015). Spectrum of retinal vascular diseases associated with paracentral acute middle maculopathy. *American Journal of Ophthalmology 160*(1), 26–34.e1. https://doi.org/10.1016/j.ajo.2015.04.004. PMID: 25849522.

Chu, Y. K., Hong, Y. T., Byeon, S. H., & Oh Woong, K. (2013). In vivo detection of acute ischemic damage in retinal arterial occlusion with optical coherence tomography: A "prominent middle limiting membrane sign." *Retina*, *33*, 2110–2117.

Coady, P. A., Cunningham, E. T., Vora, R. A., McDonald, H. R., Johnson, R. N., Jumper, J. M., et al. (2015). Spectral domain optical coherence tomography findings in eyes with acute ischaemic retinal whitening. *British Journal of Ophthalmology*, *99*, 586–592.

Ritter, M., Sacu, S., Deak, G. G., Kircher, K., Sayegh, R. G., Priente, C., et al. (2012). In vivo identification of alteration of inner neurosensory layers in branch retinal artery occlusion. *British Journal of Ophthalmology*, *96*, 201–207.

Yu, S., Pang, C. E., Gong, Y., Freund, K. B., Yannuzzi, L. A., Rahimy, E., et al. (2015). The spectrum of superficial and deep capillary ischemia in retinal artery occlusion. *American Journal of Ophthalmology*, *159*(1), 53–63.e1-2. https://doi.org/10.1016/j.ajo.2014.09.027. PMID: 25244976.

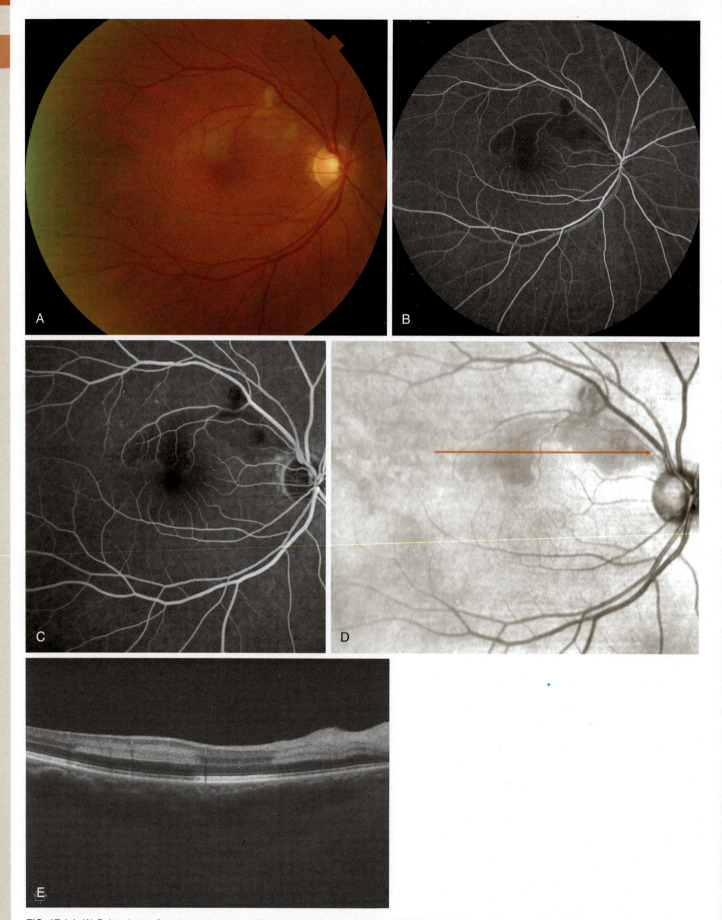

FIG. 17.1.1 (A) Color photo of acute superotemporal branch retinal artery occlusion (BRAO). (B) Fluorescein angiogram at 22 seconds shows delayed filling of the affected artery and hypoperfusion of the affected area. (C) At 2 minutes, the affected artery has filled by retrograde flow. (D) The area of the BRAO superior to the fovea is highlighted in the enface image. (E) Spectral domain OCT (Cirrus, Zeiss) reveals increased hyperreflectivity of the inner retinal and nerve fiber layers adjacent to the optic nerve. Temporal to the nerve, there is hyperreflectivity of the middle retinal layers (paracentral acute middle maculopathy) and shadowing of the deeper structures/photoreceptors.

Central Retinal Arterial Occlusion

Nadia K. Waheed | Caroline R. Baumal

17.2

Summary

Central retinal artery occlusion (CRAO) results from obstruction of the central retinal artery, which is a major branch of the ophthalmic artery. The central retinal artery provides oxygen and nutrients to the inner retina and the surface of the optic nerve. The cause of the occlusion is often embolic, but may also be thrombotic, inflammatory, traumatic, or from vasospasm. In patients over 70 years of age, giant cell arteritis is more likely to be the underlying cause than in younger patients. Risk factors include atherosclerosis, cardiac disease, coagulopathies, age range between 60 and 65 years, male gender, smoking, and diabetes mellitus. Additional risk factors include endocarditis, atrial myxoma, inflammatory diseases of the blood vessels, and predisposition to blood clots. Patients typically present with sudden, acute, painless, unilateral loss of vision. Acuity is counting fingers/hand motions in 75% to 90% of eyes at presentation. Fundoscopy reveals a central "cherry-red spot," surrounded by pale ischemic retina. The pale white color is secondary to inner retinal ischemia; the red spot is the spared central fovea, which receives its blood supply solely from the choroidal circulation. The artery can recanalize over time, and the inner edema clears with ensuing atrophy. Optic atrophy leads to permanent loss of vision. The prognosis for visual recovery is poor, and over 90% have final vision count fingers or worse. Irreversible damage to neural tissue occurs after only 90 minutes, and there is no effective treatment for embolic causes of CRAO.

Diagnosis is determined based on history and clinical features. Fluorescein angiography shows delayed central artery filling. OCT acutely reveals inner retinal thickening, hyperlucency, and loss of distinction between the inner retinal layers. Chronic CRAO shows inner retinal thinning with intact retinal pigment epithelium (RPE).

Key OCT Findings

- OCT in acute CRAO demonstrates inner retinal thickening, and the RPE, photoreceptors, and outer nuclear layer appear relatively unaffected (17.2.1).
- Chronic CRAO demonstrates inner retinal atrophy and loss of the foveal depression (Fig. 17.2.1).
- OCT angiography (OCTA) may demonstrate lack of perfusion in the retinal arteries and a generalized lack of perfusion in the retinal capillaries.

BIBLIOGRAPHY

Ahn, S. J., Woo, S. J., Park, K. H., Jung, C., Hong, J. -H., & Han, M. -H. (2015). Retinal and choroidal changes and visual outcome in central retinal artery occlusion: An optical coherence tomography study. *American Journal of Ophthalmology, 159*(4), 667–676.

Chen, H., Chen, X., Qiu, Z., Xiang, D., Chen, W., & Shi, F. (2015). Quantitative analysis of retinal layers' optical intensities on 3D optical coherence tomography for central retinal artery occlusion. *Scientific Reports, 5*, 9269. https://doi.org/10.1038/srep09269.

Kapoor, K. G., Barkmeier, A. J., & Bakri, S. J. (2015). Optical coherence tomography in retinal arterial occlusions: case series and review of the literature. *Seminars in Ophthalmology, 30*, 74–79.

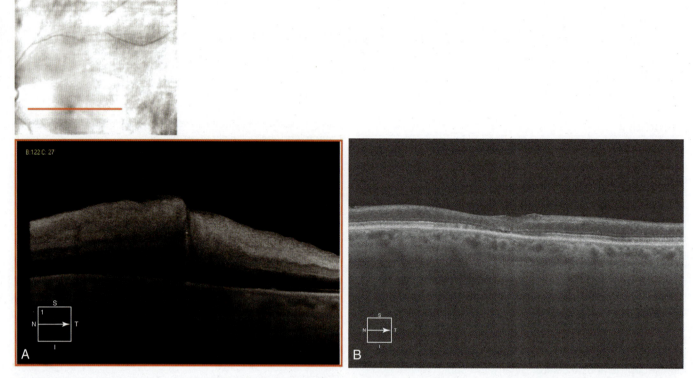

FIG. 17.2.1 (A) Inner retina thickening and hyperlucency in acute central retinal artery occlusion, shadowing the ellipsoid and choroidal details. (B) At 1 year later, there is loss of the inner retinal architecture and no distinct foveal depression. The retinal pigment epithelium remains intact.

Birdshot Retinochoroidopathy

Eduardo Uchiyama

18.1.1

Summary

Birdshot retinochoroidopathy (BSRC) is a bilateral, chronic, idiopathic inflammatory disorder that affects predominantly the retina and choroid. It is characterized by mild anterior chamber inflammation, vitritis, retinal vasculitis, and the presence of multiple hypopigmented fundus lesions. BSRC is strongly associated with human leukocyte antigen (HLA)-A29 (Fig. 18.1.1.1). OCT is the most common imaging modality used to monitor disease activity and response to treatment. Macular changes visible on OCT at presentation vary widely and include normal appearance, mild disruption of retinal architecture (Figs. 18.1.1.2–18.1.1.7), and even severely edematous or atrophic changes. Detecting and monitoring cystoid macular edema (CME) is particularly important, because this is the most common cause of decreased vision in affected patients with BSRC. OCT with enhanced depth imaging (EDI-OCT) may reveal choroidal thinning in long-standing cases, in addition to macular thinning. There is no consistent relationship between lesions seen on OCT and lesions seen clinically or on indocyanine-green angiography (ICGA). In addition to CME, other secondary features of BSRC associated with vision loss include epiretinal membrane (ERM) formation, retinal thinning, choroidal neovascular membrane (CNV), and lamellar macular hole formation. In advanced cases, diffuse retinal dysfunction can cause severe vision loss associated with retinal thinning and disruption of the inner segment/outer segment/ellipsoid zone (IS/OS/EZ) on OCT.

Key OCT Features

- CME is the most common cause of vision loss.
- Retinal thinning and disruption of the IS/OS/EZ worsen as disease progresses and correlates with vision loss.
- After successful treatment, OCT demonstrates resolution of CME and, in some patients, improvement of outer retinal changes.
- EDI-OCT is useful to best reveal choroidal thinning in long-standing cases (Figs. 18.1.1.4–18.1.1.5).
- Similar to other inflammatory chorioretinal conditions, ERM and CNV formation are sometimes manifest secondarily.

BIBLIOGRAPHY

Uchiyama, E. (2017). Birdshot retinochoroidopathy. In G. Papaliodis (Ed.), *Uveitis: A practical guide to the diagnosis and treatment of intraocular inflammation*. Geneva: Springer.

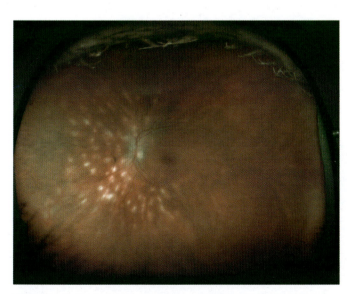

FIG. 18.1.1.1 Fundus photograph of a patient with poorly controlled birdshot retinochoroidopathy. Birdshot lesions are seen in the posterior pole along with perivascular exudation and optic disc pallor.

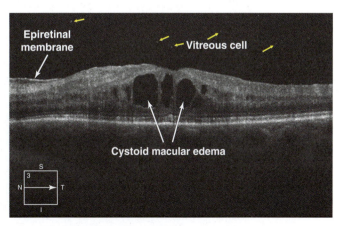

FIG. 18.1.1.2 A patient with recently diagnosed birdshot retinochoroidopathy has characteristic OCT features, including cystoid macular edema, epiretinal membrane, and vitreous cells *(yellow arrows)*.

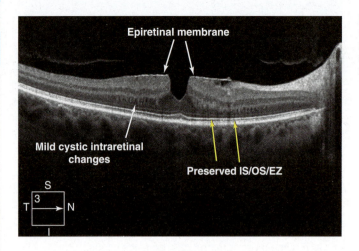

FIG. 18.1.1.3 Chronic inflammation caused epiretinal membrane formation and associated mild cystic changes in this patient with birdshot retinochoroidopathy. Note that this patient has mild/early disease and has a preserved IS/OS/EZ. *IS/OS/EZ*, Inner segment/outer segment/ellipsoid zone.

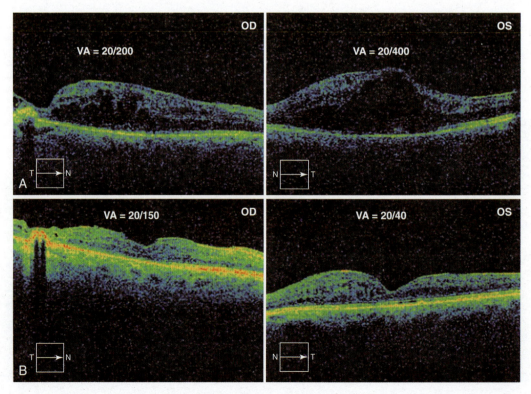

FIG. 18.1.1.4 (A) Bilateral cystoid macular edema (CME) in a patient with poorly controlled birdshot retinochoroidopathy. Visual acuity *(VA)* measured 20/200 OD and 20/400 OS. (B) At 1 year after treatment with mycophenolate mofetil, CME has mostly resolved and vision improved to 20/150 OD and 20/40 OS.

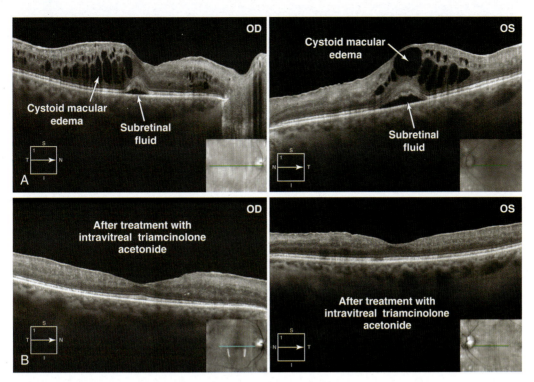

FIG. 18.1.1.5 (A) Bilateral cystoid macular edema (CME) and subretinal fluid in a patient with birdshot retinochoroidopathy. (B) At 1 month after treatment with intravitreal triamcinolone acetonide, there is brisk resolution of both CME and subretinal fluid.

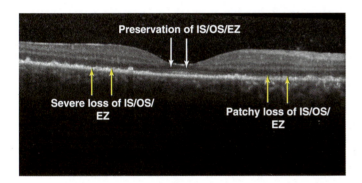

FIG. 18.1.1.6 Severe loss of IS/OS/EZ in a patient with active birdshot retinochoroidopathy. Visual acuity measured 20/40 because of preservation of the central IS/OS/EZ. *IS/OS/EZ,* Inner segment/outer segment/ellipsoid zone.

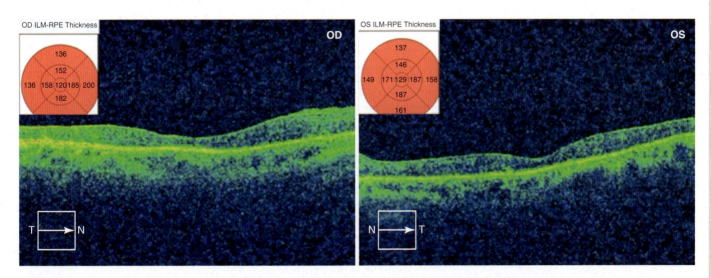

FIG. 18.1.1.7 Severe bilateral retinal thinning and atrophy in a patient with long-standing birdshot retinochoroidopathy. Visual acuity measured counting fingers at 2 feet.

Acute Posterior Multifocal Placoid Pigment Epitheliopathy

Darin R. Goldman

18.1.2

Summary

Acute posterior multifocal placoid pigment epitheliopathy (APMPPE) is a poorly understood, rare, bilateral outer retinal and/or choroidal syndrome that predominantly affects the macula. The cause is thought to be a localized inflammatory response to a recent generalized viral illness. The clinical appearance is that of a multifocal array of flat, cream-colored lesions in an inkblot or irregular pattern, usually centered on the macula. The clinical course is usually self-limited, marked by an initial acute phase followed by a resolution phase. Fluorescein angiography has a typical appearance with early hypofluorescence and late, irregular hyperfluorescence. It often shows additional lesions that are not seen clinically. OCT can provide useful information to help distinguish this entity from other similar inflammatory macular conditions. In the acute, active stage of disease, OCT shows multiple focal disruptions of the retinal pigment epithelium (RPE), inner segment/outer segment/ellipsoid zone (IS/OS/EZ), and external limiting membrane (ELM), with overlying hyperreflectivity of the outer retina limited to the outer nuclear layer and outward layers. Localized thickening of the inner retina overlying active lesions has been reported. Rarely, subretinal fluid and intraretinal fluid within the outer retinal layers may be present, similar to the appearance in Vogt-Koyanagi-Harada syndrome (see Chapter 18.2). In the resolution phase, OCT findings generally improve with reappearance of outer retinal bands along with lessening and eventual resolution of outer nuclear layer hyperreflectivity. However, permanent localized RPE irregularities and outer retinal atrophy with loss of photoreceptors may develop.

Key OCT Features

- OCT abnormalities in APMPPE correlate with clinically identifiable lesions.
- OCT findings in the acute phase show hyperreflectivity or disruption of the outer plexiform layer contiguous through to the RPE, which includes the photoreceptors (Figs. 18.1.2.1A–D and 18.1.2.2A–E).
- OCT findings in the resolution phase may normalize or leave permanent defects in the outer nuclear layer, IS/OS/EZ, and RPE (Figs. 18.1.2.1E and 18.1.2.2D–F).
- Atypical OCT findings include intraretinal fluid, significant subretinal fluid, and localized thickening of the inner retina (Fig. 18.1.2.3).

BIBLIOGRAPHY

Goldenberg, D., Habot-Wilner, Z., Loewenstein, A., Goldstein, M. (2012). Spectral domain optical coherence tomography classification of acute posterior multifocal placoid pigment epitheliopathy. *Retina 32*(7), 1403–1410.

Querques, G., Querques, L., Bux, A. V., Iaculli, C., & Delle Noci, N. (2010). High-definition OCT findings in acute posterior multifocal placoid pigment epitheliopathy. *Ophthalmic Surgery, Lasers and Imaging Retina 41*, e1–e6.

Scheufele, T. A., Witkin, A. J., Schocket, L. S., et al. (2005). Photoreceptor atrophy in acute posterior multifocal placoid pigment epitheliopathy demonstrated by optical coherence tomography. *Retina 25*(8), 1109–1112.

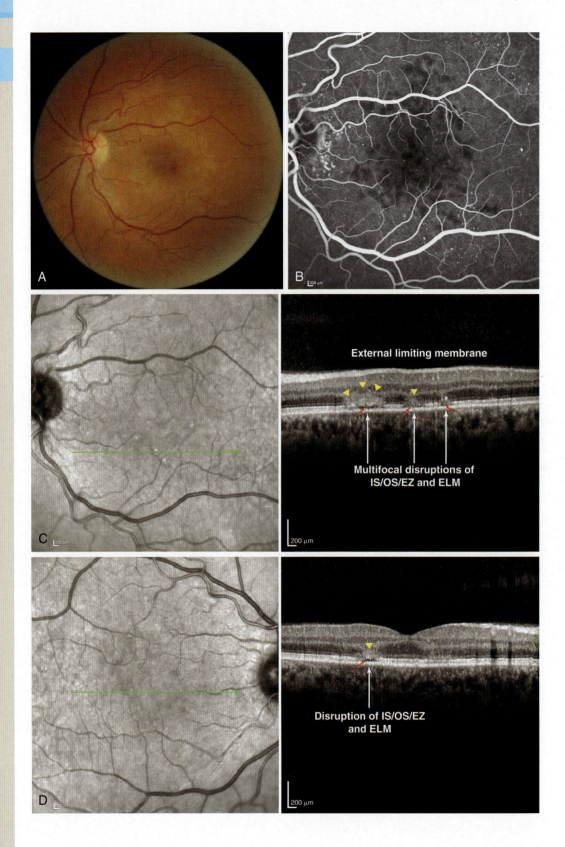

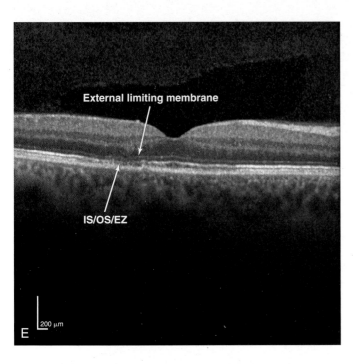

FIG. 18.1.2.1 Typical clinical appearance (A) and fluorescein angiography (B) of acute posterior multifocal placoid pigment epitheliopathy at presentation. (C) Corresponding OCT in the acute phase shows multifocal areas of disrupted IS/OS/EZ and ELM bands with abnormal hyperreflectivity of the outer retina *(arrowheads)* spanning from the outer plexiform layer to the retinal pigment epithelium, inclusive of the photoreceptors. There is faint subretinal fluid associated with each lesion *(red arrows)*. (D) The fellow eye shows similar findings. (E) At 2 weeks after presentation, OCT shows near normalization of the outer retinal architecture with a restored ELM and IS/OS/EZ band, although they remain attenuated. *ELM*, External limiting membrane; *IS/OS/EZ*, inner segment/outer segment/ellipsoid zone. (Courtesy Robin A. Vora, MD, and John Lewis, MD.)

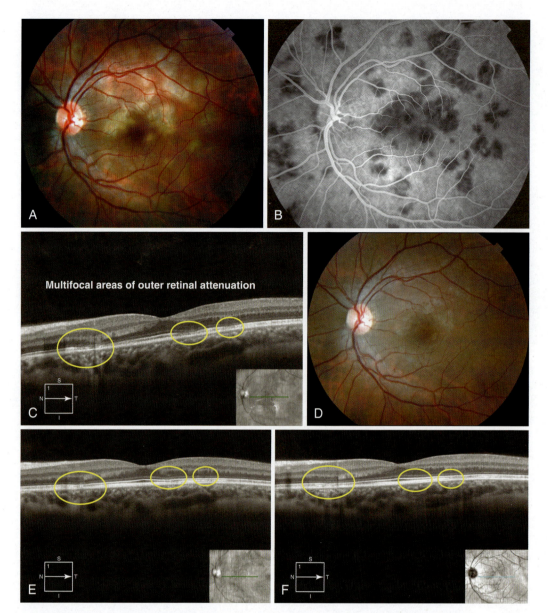

FIG. 18.1.2.2 At presentation in the subacute phase of acute posterior multifocal placoid pigment epitheliopathy, numerous lesions are visible clinically (A) and many more visible angiographically (B). OCT shows multifocal areas of outer retinal attenuation *(yellow circles)* affecting predominantly the photoreceptors and retinal pigment epithelium (RPE), with relative sparing of the outer nuclear layer (C). 6 months later, the active lesions are resolved (D), leaving pigment clumping at the level of the RPE with a nearly complete normalization of the OCT appearance, although faint inner segment/outer segment/ellipsoid zone attenuation remains (E). This normalization trend continues for 1 year (F). Note that the same areas highlighted by *yellow circles* in panels C, E, and F. (Panels A and B with permission from Reichel, E., Duker, J., Goldman D., Vora R., & Fein, J. (2015). Handbook of retinal disease. London: JP Medical.)

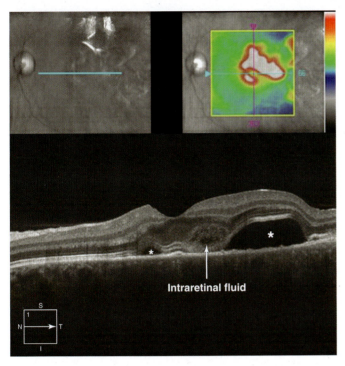

FIG. 18.1.2.3 Atypical case of acute posterior multifocal placoid pigment epitheliopathy shows significant subretinal fluid *(asterisks)* and localized cystic thickening of the outer retina. These features can resemble findings in Vogt-Koyanagi-Harada syndrome.

Multiple Evanescent White Dot Syndrome | 18.1.3

Darin R. Goldman | Nora W. Muakkassa

Summary

Multiple evanescent white dot syndrome (MEWDS) is thought to be an inflammatory outer retinal disease that occurs in young, myopic women. A flulike prodrome may occur, with symptoms including photopsias, blurred vision, or scotomas. Findings on examination may include mild vitreous cells, mild disc edema, foveal granularity, and small white dots at the level of the deep retina. Visual field testing may reveal an enlarged blind spot. Fluorescein angiography typically shows early wreath-like hyperfluorescence with late staining. Indocyanine green angiography reveals hypocyanescent spots that are usually more numerous than the white spots noted on examination. OCT shows areas of disruption of the inner segment/outer segment/ellipsoid zone (IS/OS/EZ) throughout the posterior pole (Figs. 18.1.3.1 and 18.1.3.2). These areas of disruption are more diffuse than the focal white dots on funduscopic examination. Posterior vitreous cells also may be visible on OCT imaging. OCT findings typically normalize spontaneously over time as symptoms abate and white dots resolve.

Key OCT Features

- Acute findings include disruption of the IS/OS/EZ.
- Inflammatory cells in the posterior vitreous, seen as hyper-reflective dots, may be seen during the acute phase.
- IS/OS disruption is diffuse and does not necessarily correlate with white dots seen clinically.
- The IS/OS/EZ typically regains a normal appearance over several months, although mild IS/OS abnormalities may persist.

BIBLIOGRAPHY

Li, D., & Kishi, S. (2009). Restored photoreceptor outer segment damage in multiple evanescent white dot syndrome. *Ophthalmology, 116,* 762–770.

Silva, R. A., Albini, T. A., & Flynn, H. W., Jr. (2012). Multiple evanescent white dot syndromes. *Journal of Ophthalmic Inflammation and Infection, 2,* 109–111.

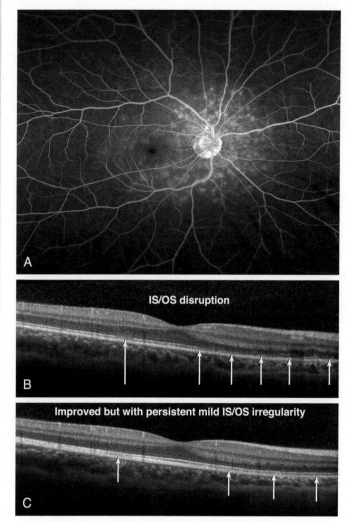

FIG. 18.1.3.1 Multiple evanescent white dot syndrome. (A) Late phase fluorescein angiogram reveals stippled hyperfluorescence. (B) OCT at presentation demonstrates disruption of the IS/OS/ellipsoid zone temporal and nasal to the fovea. (C) OCT 6 months later shows a trend toward normalization of the IS/OS appearance, although mild attenuation persists. *IS/OS*, Inner segment/outer segment. (Images courtesy of Trexler Topping, MD.)

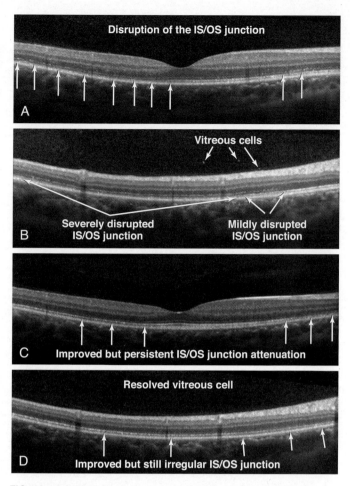

FIG. 18.1.3.2 Multiple evanescent white dot syndrome. (A) OCT at presentation shows diffuse disruption of the IS/OS/ellipsoid zone (EZ). (B) OCT through the inferior macula shows diffuse IS/OS disruption and inflammatory cells in the posterior vitreous, which appear as hyperreflective dots. (C) At 4 months later, OCT shows improved but persistent IS/OS attenuation. (D) At 6 months after presentation, OCT through the inferior macula shows resolved vitreous cells and restoration of the IS/OS/EZ, though mild irregularity persists. *IS/OS*, Inner segment/ outer segment. (Courtesy Jeffrey Heier, MD.)

Summary

Serpiginous choroiditis is an inflammatory condition of the choroid that affects the outer retina and the retinal pigment epithelium (RPE). The cause is unknown, although tuberculosis should be ruled out in all cases. The clinical course is marked by progression, regression, and recurrences. The affected eye(s) typically has a characteristic unifocal, serpentine, grayish lesion located beneath the retina, typically in a peripapillary or macular location. Over time, the active lesion regresses, leaving generalized atrophy of the RPE and underlying choriocapillaris. Recurrent lesions typically initiate at the edges of old inactive areas. Vision loss occurs as a result of atrophy underlying the fovea or secondary choroidal neovascularization.

OCT features of active lesions include hyperreflectivity and thickening of the outer retina. Homogeneous hyperreflective subretinal material accumulation also may occur. OCT features of inactive lesions include generalized atrophy of the outer retina and RPE. Enhanced-depth OCT imaging may be useful to detect choroidal ischemia associated with active lesions, which should resolve with resolution of active disease.

Key OCT Features

- Active lesions feature homogeneous hyperreflectivity of the very outer retina that coalesces with similar subretinal material and the underlying RPE (Fig. 18.1.4.1).
- Inactive lesions show generalized outer retinal and RPE atrophy. Subretinal fibrosis also may be present (Fig. 18.1.4.2).

BIBLIOGRAPHY

Carreño, E., Fernandez-Sanz, G., Sim, D. A., Keane, P. A., Westcott, M. C., Tufail, A., et al. (2015). Multimodal imaging of macular serpiginous choroidopathy from acute presentation to quiescence. *Ophthalmic Surgery, Lasers & Imaging Retina*, 46(2), 266–270.

Lim, W. K., Buggage, R. R., & Nussenblatt, R. B. (2005). Serpiginous choroiditis. *Survey of Ophthalmology*, 50(3), 231–244.

Punjabi, O. S., Rich, R., Davis, J. L., Gregori, G., Flynn, H. W., Jr, et al., Lujan, B. J., et al. (2008). Imaging serpiginous choroidopathy with spectral domain optical coherence tomography. *Ophthalmic Surgery, Lasers & Imaging*, 39(4 suppl), S95–S98.

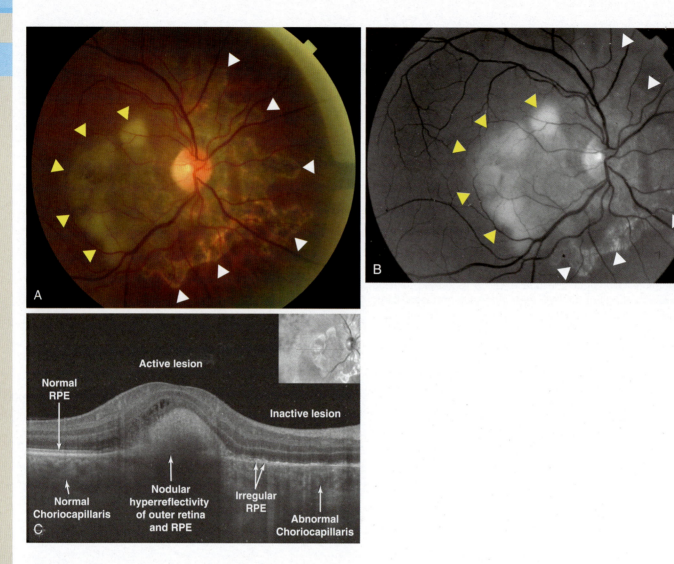

FIG. 18.1.4.1 Acute serpiginous choroiditis. (A and B) Color and red-free photographs show active choroiditis *(yellow arrowheads)* in the macula emanating from older, inactive lesions that exhibit RPE and choriocapillaris atrophy *(white arrowheads)*. (C) OCT shows two distinct abnormal areas: (1) acute lesion exhibits a nodular elevation of hyperreflective material infiltrating the outer retina with obliteration of the underlying RPE and (2) inactive lesion exhibits irregular RPE and underlying choriocapillaris. *RPE*, Retinal pigment epithelium.

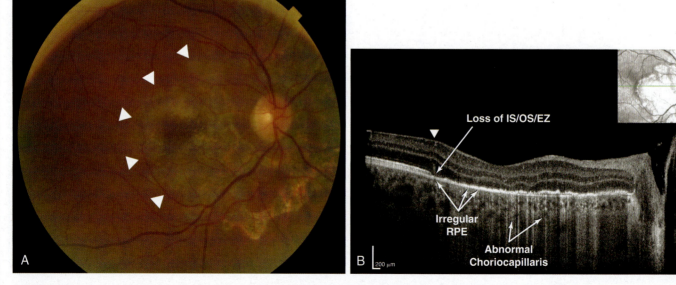

FIG. 18.1.4.2 At 1 week after systemic prednisone. (A) Color photograph shows disappearance of the subretinal white infiltrate (see Fig. 18.1.4.1) that is replaced by developing atrophy of the RPE and choriocapillaris. (B) In the area of the previously active lesion, OCT shows loss of the inner segment/outer segment/ellipsoid zone *(IS/OS/EZ)* with outer retinal atrophy, diffuse RPE irregularity with dropout, and an abnormal choriocapillaris. Note that unaffected retina/choroid is located to the left of the *arrowhead*. *RPE*, Retinal pigment epithelium.

Summary

Multifocal choroiditis and panuveitis (MCP) and punctuate inner choroidopathy (PIC) are idiopathic inflammatory disorders that primarily affect the outer retina and subretinal pigment epithelium (RPE) bilaterally (Spaide et al., 2013). The two conditions exhibit many similarities and are considered within a spectrum of the same disorder, with PIC being a subtype of MCP. Younger myopic females are typically affected. MCP exhibits vitreous inflammation during active disease, whereas PIC typically lacks intraocular inflammation. Active lesions appear as yellowish or gray circular subretinal irregularities. Inactive lesions appear as multifocal "punched-out" atrophic areas with pigmented borders located throughout the fundus that can resemble those seen in presumed ocular histoplasmosis syndrome.

Secondary choroidal neovascularization (CNV) formation is the most frequent cause of vision loss. The distinction between inflammatory lesion and CNV is critical but can be difficult, even with fluorescein angiography. OCT, particularly OCT angiography, is extremely helpful in differentiating between these two pathologic sequelae (Figs. 18.1.5.1–18.1.5.7). Treatment includes systemic immunosuppression, localized treatment to inflammatory lesions (steroid), and CNV (anti–vascular endothelial growth factor [anti-VEGF]). Treatment response, best monitored by OCT, can help confirm the type of underlying active lesion.

Key OCT Features

- Acute inflammatory lesions can best be differentiated from CNVs using OCT angiography, particularly when fluorescein angiography is inconclusive (Figs. 18.1.5.3 and 18.1.5.7).
- Both inflammatory lesions and CNVs affect the outer retinal layers and sub-RPE space, exhibiting mixed reflectivity with dehiscence of the RPE layer. The inner segment/outer segment/ellipsoid zone is often absent.
- CNV tend to be less well defined than inflammatory lesions and often have associated subretinal fluid.
- Chronic or inactive lesions are well-defined hyperreflective nodular elevations of the RPE with overlying layers intact and visible.

REFERENCE

Spaide, R. F., Goldberg, N., & Freund, K. B. (2013). Redefining multifocal choroiditis and panuveitis and punctate inner choroidopathy through multimodal imaging. *Retina 33*(7), 1315–1324.

BIBLIOGRAPHY

Cheng, L., Chen, X., Weng, S., Gong, Y., Yu, S., Xu, X. (2016). Spectral-domain optical coherence tomography angiography findings in multifocal choroiditis with active lesions. *American Journal of Ophthalmology*, *169*, 145–161.

Levison, A. L., Baynes, K. M., Lowder, C. Y., Kaiser, P. K., & Srivastava, S. K. (2017). Choroidal neovascularisation on optical coherence tomography angiography in punctate innerchoroidopathy and multifocal choroiditis. *British Journal of Ophthalmology 101*(5), 616–622. https://doi.org/10.1136/bjophthalmol-2016-308806.

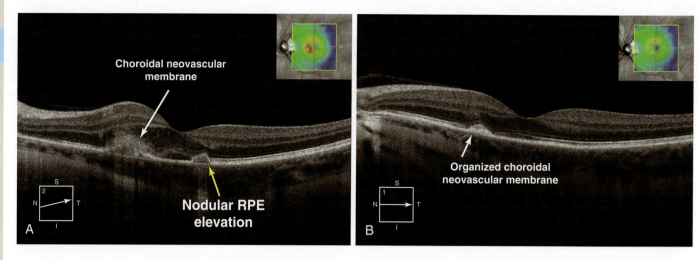

FIG. 18.1.5.1 (A) Multifocal choroiditis and panuveitis with active choroidal neovascularization (CNV). There are two separate elevated lesions located beneath the RPE. The nasal lesion *(white arrow)* is ill-defined, with loss of the RPE layer and an abnormal subretinal hyperreflective signal extending into the outer retinal layers. This area corresponds to a CNV with associated leakage on fluorescein angiography. The temporal lesion *(yellow arrow)* is a well-defined nodular sub-RPE elevation with medium reflectivity. This area did not have any definitive corresponding leakage on fluorescein angiography, suggesting no CNV. Subretinal fluid is also present (between white and yellow arrows). (B) After treatment with anti–vascular endothelial growth factor therapy, the temporal lesion regressed completely and the nasal lesion organized into a well-defined hyperreflective dome-shaped elevation at the level of the RPE. *RPE*, Retinal pigment epithelium. (Courtesy Patrick E. Rubsamen, MD, and Eduardo Uchiyama, MD.)

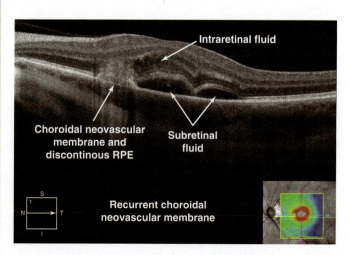

FIG. 18.1.5.2 At 3 months after initial anti–vascular endothelial growth factor therapy, the patient had recurrence active choroidal neovascularization with an appearance similar to the initial occurrence (see Fig. 18.1.5.1). Note that the RPE is discontinuous and there is both intraretinal and subretinal fluid. *RPE*, Retinal pigment epithelium. (Courtesy Patrick E. Rubsamen, MD, and Eduardo Uchiyama, MD.)

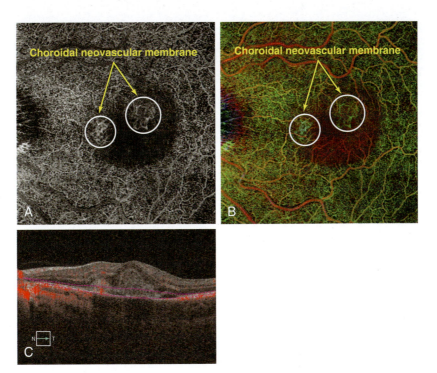

FIG. 18.1.5.3 Multifocal choroiditis and panuveitis with active choroidal neovascularization. OCT angiography slabs show two distinct areas of choroidal neovascularization *(circles)* located within the deep retinal slab. Corresponding OCT B-scan is shown with segmentation lines that demarcate the OCT angiography slabs *(bottom).* (Courtesy Patrick E. Rubsamen, MD, and Eduardo Uchiyama, MD.)

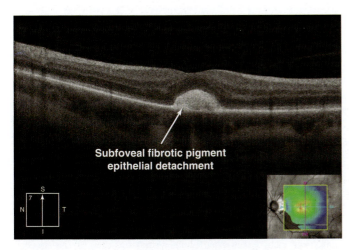

FIG. 18.1.5.4 At 6 months after initial presentation, despite anti–vascular endothelial growth factor treatment, a subfoveal fibrotic pigment epithelial detachment developed, with visual acuity measuring counting fingers. (Courtesy Patrick E. Rubsamen, MD, and Eduardo Uchiyama, MD.)

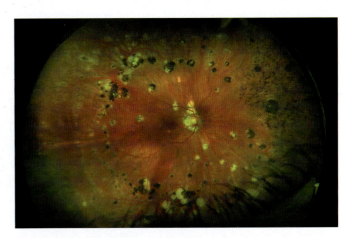

FIG. 18.1.5.5 Wide-field fundus image of multifocal choroiditis and panuveitis illustrating numerous atrophic and pigmented round lesions distributed throughout the fundus. (Courtesy Patrick E. Rubsamen, MD, and Eduardo Uchiyama, MD.)

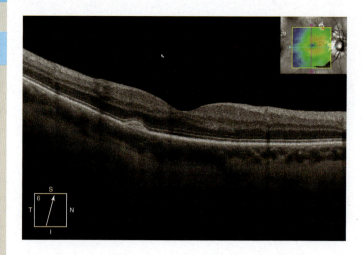

FIG. 18.1.5.6 Baseline OCT in a patient with inactive multifocal choroiditis. (Courtesy Patrick E. Rubsamen, MD, and Eduardo Uchiyama, MD.)

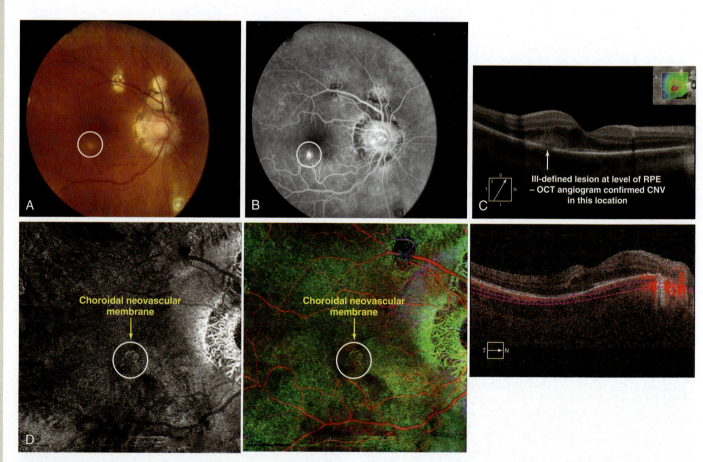

Ill-defined lesion at level of RPE – OCT angiogram confirmed CNV in this location

Choroidal neovascular membrane

Choroidal neovascular membrane

FIG. 18.1.5.7 (A) Color photograph of an active macular lesion *(circle)* in multifocal choroiditis and panuveitis. (B) Fluorescein angiogram reveals hyperfluorescence of the lesion resulting from staining but no definitive leakage, which was inconclusive regarding the presence of CNV. (C) Structural *OCT* B-scan shows an ill-defined, moderately reflective lesion at the level of the *RPE* with obscuration of the outer retinal layers. (D) OCT angiogram slabs confirm the presence of CNV in this location *(circle)*. A corresponding OCT B-scan is shown with segmentation lines that demarcate the OCT angiography slab *(bottom)*. *CNV*, Choroidal neovascularization; *RPE*, retinal pigment epithelium. (Courtesy Patrick E. Rubsamen, MD, and Eduardo Uchiyama, MD.)

Vogt-Koyanagi-Harada Disease

Darin R. Goldman

18.2

Summary

Vogt-Koyanagi-Harada (VKH) disease is a multiphase (prodromal, acute, convalescent, and chronic recurrent phases) systemic condition that manifests with vestibular-cochlear symptoms including hearing loss and tinnitus, dermatologic signs including vitiligo, and prominent posterior segment findings including bilateral uveitis, serous retinal detachment, and choroidal inflammation. In addition to fluorescein angiography and indocyanine green angiography, OCT has proved useful as an imaging modality to aid in the diagnosis of VKH disease and monitor response to systemic treatment. In the acute phase, OCT reveals characteristic serous retinal detachments (subretinal fluid) and choroidal thickening (Figs. 18.2.1 and 18.2.2). These findings correlate with active disease and, in the convalescent phase, subretinal fluid resolves and choroidal thickness decreases, both features that can be used to monitor treatment response. Reduction of focal hyperreflectivity of the inner choroid in acute and convalescent stages of VKH disease may correlate with choroidal inflammation/infiltration and account for compromising choriocapillaris blood flow (Fong et al., 2011) (Figs. 18.2.3 and 18.2.4). Additional OCT features of VKH disease include subretinal septae, retinal pigment epithelium (RPE)/choroidal folds, and intraretinal cysts in various layers of the outer retina. These additional features help distinguish VKH disease from central serous chorioretinopathy (see Chapter 8.1).

Key OCT Features

- The presence and height of subretinal fluid and choroidal thickness on OCT correlate with disease activity and visual acuity, which can be useful to gauge treatment response.
- Subretinal septae and RPE/choroidal folds are distinguishing features of VKH that are well visualized on OCT (Fig. 18.2.2).
- Intraretinal fluid may be present in the outer retinal layers.
- OCT features normalize with time (Fig. 18.2.5).

REFERENCE

Fong, A. H., Li, K. K., & Wong, D. (2011). Choroidal evaluation using enhanced depth imaging spectral-domain optical coherence tomography in Vogt-Koyanagi-Harada disease. *Retina*, *31*(3), 502–509.

BIBLIOGRAPHY

O'Keefe, G. A., & Rao, N. A. (2017). Vogt-Koyanagi-Harada disease. *Surveys in Ophthalmology*, *62*(1), 1–25.

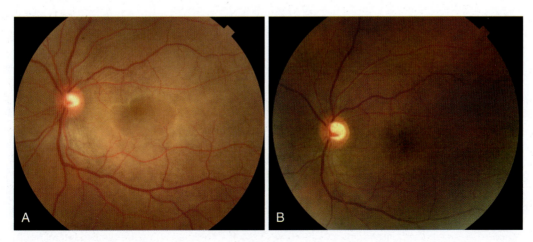

FIG. 18.2.1 (A) Vogt-Koyanagi-Harada disease in the acute stage with visible serous retinal detachment in the macula and surrounding chorioretinal folds. (B) At 1 month after treatment with high-dose systemic prednisone, there is near complete resolution.

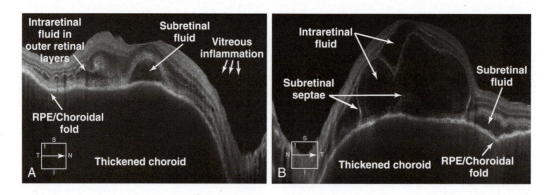

FIG. 18.2.2 Right (A) and left (B) eyes in the acute stage of Vogt-Koyanagi-Harada (VKH) disease show significant intraretinal fluid accumulation located within the outer retina. Additional characteristic OCT features of VKH that are illustrated include intraretinal and subretinal fluid, subretinal septae, a thickened choroid, RPE/choroidal folds, and vitreous inflammation. *RPE*, Retinal pigment epithelium.

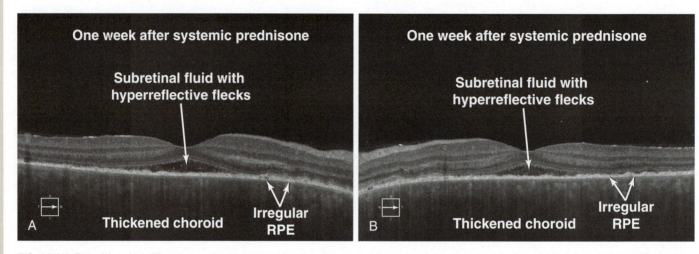

FIG. 18.2.3 Right (A) and left (B) eyes 1 week after treatment with systemic prednisone. There is dramatic reduction of active disease features on OCT. Subretinal fluid and choroidal thickness are both reduced from baseline but remain abnormal. Hyperreflective flecks are seen within the subretinal fluid, and the RPE retains an irregular contour. *RPE*, Retinal pigment epithelium.

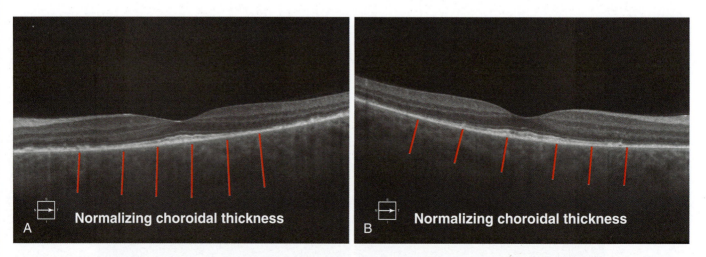

FIG. 18.2.4 Right (A) and left (B) eyes 1 month after treatment, in the convalescent phase. Subretinal fluid has completely resolved. The retinal pigment epithelium still has an irregular contour that has improved. The choroidal thickness is near normal; its depth can be visualized in certain areas (estimated by *red bars*).

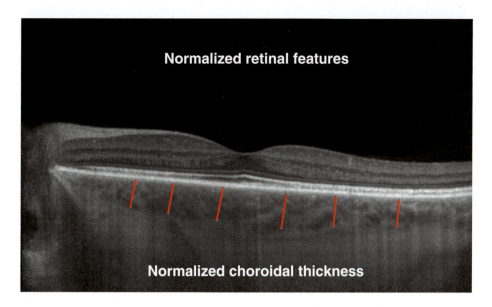

FIG. 18.2.5 At 1 year after treatment, all OCT features of disease have resolved. The retinal pigment epithelium has a regained a linear contour, and the choroidal thickness has normalized (*red arrows*).

Darin R. Goldman | Nora W. Muakkassa

Summary

Sympathetic ophthalmia is a rare, bilateral, granulomatous uveitis resulting from autoantibodies targeting ocular tissues after penetrating injury or surgery. Findings range from mild anterior uveitis to severe panuveitis. Additional clinical findings include mutton-fat keratic precipitates, vitritis, papillitis, and serous retinal detachments. Dalen-Fuchs nodules are a classic finding present in only 25% to 35% of cases. These nodules are composed of subretinal retinal pigment epithelium (RPE) epithelioid cells. OCT findings include focal nodular hyperreflective lesions at the level of the RPE, which correspond clinically with Dalen-Fuchs nodules (Fig. 18.3.1). Additionally, there may be diffuse external limiting membrane (ELM) and inner segment/outer segment/ellipsoid zone (IS/OS/EZ) loss. Subretinal fluid and choroidal thickening may be present in cases with serous retinal detachment. After treatment, which typically includes systemic immunosuppression, these findings often resolve. However, attenuated areas of the IS/OS/EZ and ELM may persist (Fig. 18.3.2).

Key OCT Findings

- Dalen-Fuchs nodules are hyperreflective nodular lesions at the level of the RPE.
- Diffuse losses of the ELM and IS/OS/EZ are common, along with serous retinal detachment and a thickened choroid, all of which should improve after treatment.
- Permanent irregularities of the IS/OS/EZ and ELM may persist.

BIBLIOGRAPHY

Behdad, B., Rahmani, S., Montahaei, T., Soheilian, R., & Soheilian, M. (2015). Enhanced depth imaging OCT (EDI-OCT) findings in acute phase of sympathetic ophthalmia. *International Ophthalmology*, 35, 433–439.

Gupta, V., Gupta, A., Dogra, M. R., & Singh, I. (2011). Reversible retinal changes in the acute stage of sympathetic ophthalmia seen on spectral domain optical coherence tomography. *International Ophthalmology 31*, 105–110.

Muakkassa, N. W., & Witkin, A. J. (2014). Spectral-domain optical coherence tomography of sympathetic ophthalmia with Dalen-Fuchs nodules. *Ophthalmic Surgery, Lasers, & Imaging Retina, 45*(6), 610–612.

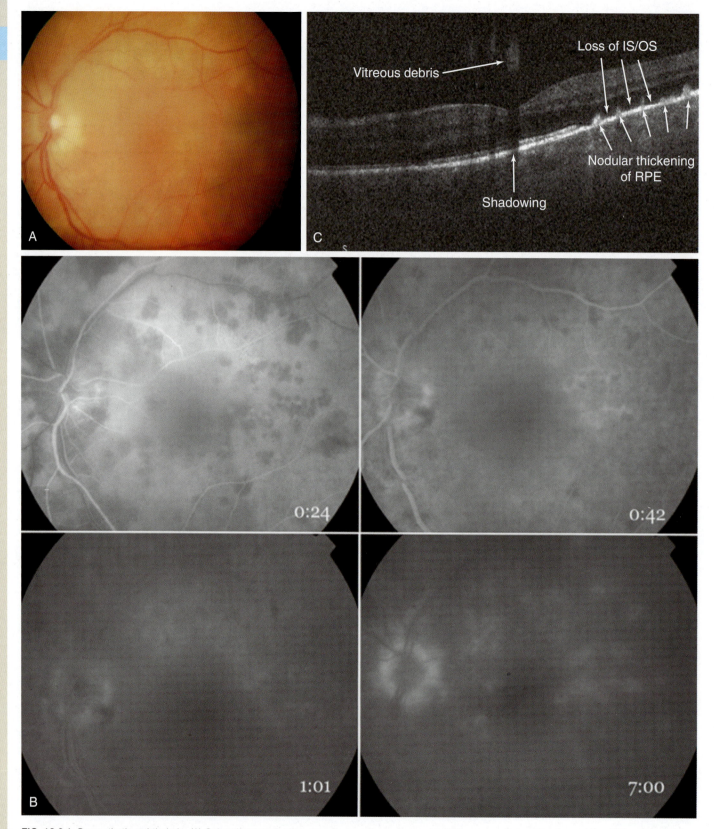

FIG. 18.3.1 Sympathetic ophthalmia. (A) Color photograph shows media opacity secondary to vitritis, peripapillary whitening, and multiple subretinal, white, creamy lesions. (B) Fluorescein angiogram shows early blockage and late staining of the peripapillary area and multiple lesions throughout the posterior pole. (C) OCT shows shadowing secondary to vitritis, hyperreflective, nodular deposits at the level of the RPE, and loss of the IS/OS/ellipsoid zone and external limiting membrane. *IS/OS*, Inner segment/outer segment; *RPE*, retinal pigment epithelium. (From Muakkassa, N. W., & Witkin, A. J. (2014). Spectral-domain optical coherence tomography of sympathetic ophthalmia with Dalen-Fuchs nodules. Ophthalmic Surgery, Lasers, & Imaging Retina. 45(6), 610–612. Reproduced with permission of SLACK Inc.)

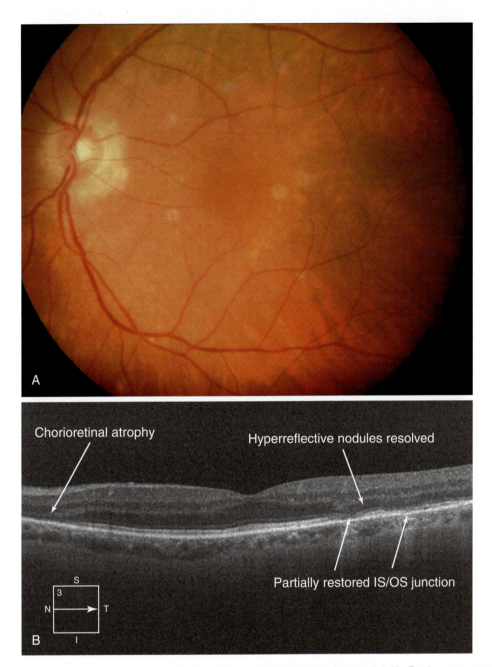

FIG. 18.3.2 Ten months after immunosuppressive therapy. (A) Color fundus photograph shows improved vitritis. Previous creamy, white, subretinal lesions have resolved, leaving scattered areas of chorioretinal atrophy. (B) OCT reveals resolved hyperreflective nodules along with a partially restored IS/OS/ellipsoid zone temporally. An area of chorioretinal atrophy is visible nasally. *IS/OS,* Inner segment/outer segment.

Toxoplasmic Chorioretinitis

19.1

Darin R. Goldman

Summary

Toxoplasmic chorioretinitis, caused by infection of the parasite *Toxoplasma gondii*, is the most common identifiable cause for posterior uveitis and focal retinitis. The clinical appearance is that of focal yellow or white retinitis with overlying vitreous inflammation. The active area of retinitis is typically adjacent to a darkly pigmented chorioretinal scar, indicative of old disease. The diagnosis of toxoplasmic chorioretinitis is usually determined based on the clinical appearance alone. Unusual cases may be difficult to differentiate from other causes of retinitis. In these cases, additional diagnostic testing, such as serology or aqueous sampling for polymerase chain reaction, may be helpful. OCT, although not definitive in its diagnostic specificity for toxoplasmic chorioretinitis, can elucidate unique findings that support the diagnosis (Figs. 19.1.1–19.1.4).

Key OCT Features

- Full-thickness retinal hyperreflectivity is present in focal areas of retinitis with distinct margins (Fig. 19.1.2).
- White spots in vitreous and within retina can be seen.
- Subretinal fluid may be present, usually only detectable via OCT.
- Round, hyperreflective plaques overlying retinal blood vessels may be seen throughout the fundus, which are strongly suggestive of toxoplasmosis chorioretinitis.

BIBLIOGRAPHY

Saito, M., Barbazetto, I. A., & Spaide, R. F. (2013). Intravitreal cellular infiltrate imaged as punctate spots by spectral-domain optical coherence tomography in eyes with posterior segment inflammatory disease. *Retina 33*(3), 559–565.

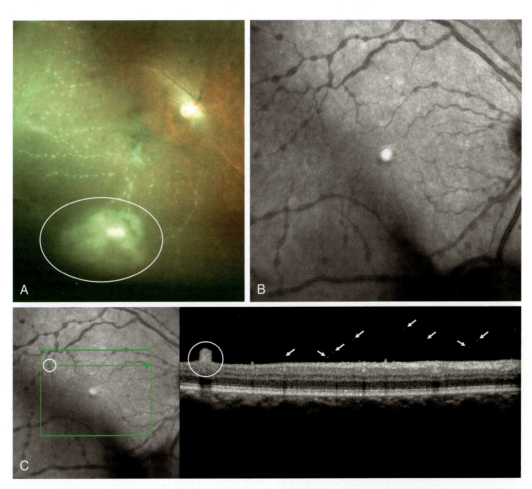

FIG. 19.1.1 (A) Diffuse toxoplasmic chorioretinitis with a large area of focal retinitis *(circle)*. (B) Infrared image highlighting spheroid plaques located on both arterioles and venules. (C) OCT in an area not involved with focal retinitis. Secondary features of active inflammation are present, including visible white blood cells in the vitreous cavity *(arrows)* and a typical perivascular spheroid deposit in cross section *(circle)*.

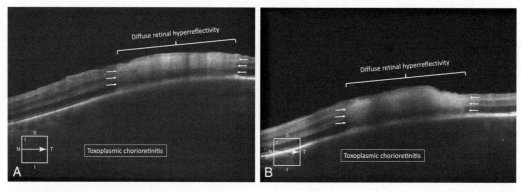

FIG. 19.1.2 (A and B) Diffuse retinal hyperreflectivity is present in a focal area of active retinitis due to toxoplasmosis *(arrows)*. The margins of involved and uninvolved retina are distinct.

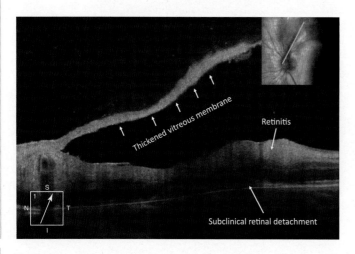

FIG. 19.1.3 Peripapillary toxoplasmic chorioretinitis. There is a highly reflective, thickened vitreous membrane due to localized inflammation. A subclinical retinal detachment is present, but difficult to appreciate. The involved area of focal retinitis is partially obscured by overlying inflammation, which causes shadowing.

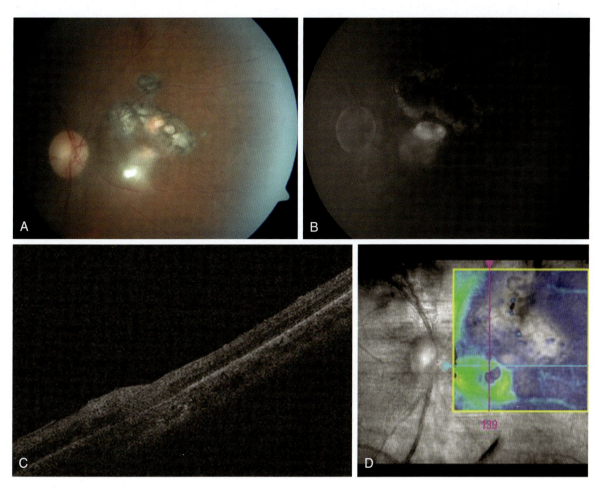

FIG. 19.1.4 (A) Color photograph and (B) fluorescein angiogram of typical toxoplasmic chorioretinitis showing an active lesion adjacent to a scar. (C and D) OCT through the area of active retinitis shows full-thickness involvement with diffuse hyperreflectivity. (Courtesy Lana Rifkin, MD.)

Acute Syphilitic Posterior Placoid Chorioretinitis

Darin R. Goldman

Summary

Syphilis is a rare cause of infectious uveitis caused by the spirochete *Treponema pallidum* that occurs in the secondary or tertiary stages of disease. Ocular involvement typically manifests as posterior uveitis with chorioretinitis. A distinctive form of this condition is termed "acute syphilitic posterior placoid chorioretinitis" (ASPPC), which exhibits a characteristic clinical appearance. Single or multiple, round, yellowish lesions within the macula, which involve the outer retina and retinal pigment epithelium (RPE), are present in one or both eyes. Although the clinical and angiographic appearance of ASPPC can be fairly distinct, OCT findings can increase diagnostic certainty in the appropriate clinical context. Distinct OCT features are present in the outer retinal and RPE layers, which typically resolve completely on appropriate antibiotic treatment (Figs. 19.2.1–19.2.3).

Key OCT Features

- In the acute phase of ASPPC, there may be shallow subretinal fluid in the fovea, which is transient, and only detectable by OCT.
- The most distinctive feature of ASPPC is patchy disruption of the inner segment/outer statement/ellipsoid zone (IS/OS/EZ)

with intermixed hyperreflective nodular lesions, which may represent thickened RPE (Fig. 19.2.1).

- The external limiting membrane is typically disrupted focally over the nodular lesions and punctate hyperreflectivity in the choroid may be present.
- With appropriate and timely treatment, abnormal OCT findings parallel clinical findings and show dramatic, complete resolution within 1 to 2 months in the majority of cases (Fig. 19.2.2).

BIBLIOGRAPHY

Burkholder, B. M., Leung, T. G., Ostheimer, T. A., Butler, N. J., Thorne, J. E., Dunn, J. P. (2014). Spectral domain optical coherence tomography findings in acute syphilitic posterior placoid chorioretinitis. *Journal of Ophthalmic Inflammation and Infection* 4(1), 2.

Eandi, C. M., Neri, P., Adelman, R. A., Yannuzzi, L. A., Cunningham, E. T., Jr, & the International Syphilis Study Group, (2012). Acute syphilitic posterior placoid chorioretinitis: report of a case series and comprehensive review of the literature. *Retina* 32(9), 1915–1941.

Pichi, F., Ciardella, A. P., Cunningham, E. T., Jr, et al., Morara, M., Veronese, C., Jumper, J. M., et al. (2014). Spectral domain optical coherence tomography findings in patients with acute syphilitic posterior placoid chorioretinopathy. *Retina* 34(2), 373–384.

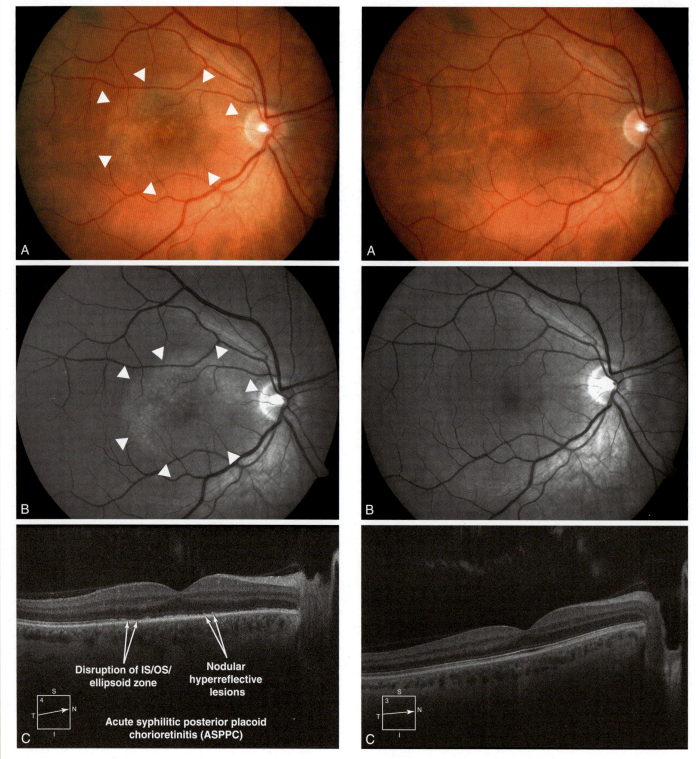

FIG. 19.2.1 (A and B) Color and red-free photographs of typical acute syphilitic posterior placoid chorioretinitis at presentation with visual acuity of 20/100. The borders of the lesion are illustrated with *arrowheads*. (C) OCT reveals characteristic patchy loss of the IS/OS/ellipsoid zone along with hyperreflective nodular retinal pigment epithelium lesions. *ASPPC*, Acute syphilitic posterior placoid chorioretinitis; *IS/OS*, inner segment/outer statement. (Courtesy Lana Rifkin, MD.)

FIG. 19.2.2 (A and B) Color and red-free photographs 1 month after intravenous ceftriaxone therapy with return of visual acuity to 20/20. (C) OCT shows normalization of the inner segment/outer statement/ellipsoid zone and resolution of the hyperreflective nodular retinal pigment epithelium lesions. (Courtesy of Lana Rifkin, MD.)

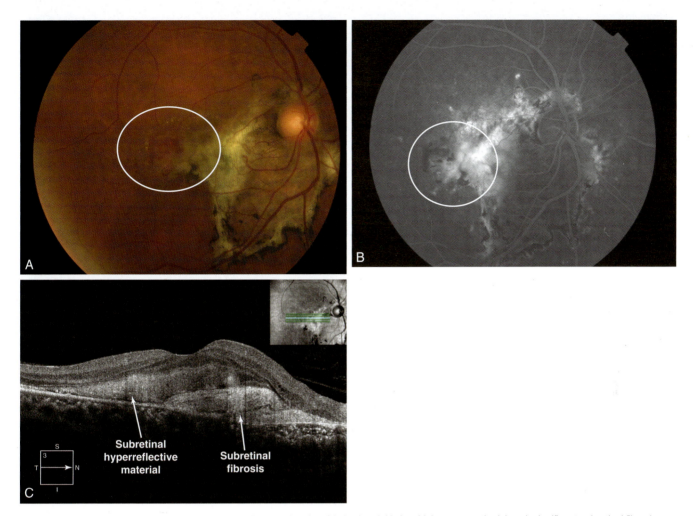

FIG. 19.2.3 (A and B) In severe cases of acute syphilitic posterior placoid chorioretinitis in which treatment is delayed, significant subretinal fibrosis can develop. In this example, a secondary choroidal neovascular membrane developed *(circle)* on the temporal edge of old scarring many years following the acute episode. (C) OCT reveals two distinct subretinal pathologic processes: subretinal hyperreflective material resulting from choroidal neovascularization and subretinal fibrosis secondary to scarring.

Summary

Mycobacterium tuberculosis is a common cause of infectious uveitis in certain tropical countries. Choroidal granuloma, chorioretinitis, and various forms of uveitis all can be ocular manifestations of tuberculosis. Involvement of the choroid can be localized or multifocal, mimicking various noninfectious ocular conditions, such as serpiginous choroiditis. Secondary abnormalities may develop within the subretinal space. OCT is particularly useful in identifying both subretinal and choroidal manifestations of tuberculosis (Figs. 19.3.1 and 19.3.2).

Key OCT Features

- Choroidal infiltration results in homogeneous hyporeflective material present beneath the retinal pigment epithelium (RPE) in a dome-shaped configuration.
- Overlying subretinal fluid may be present acutely.
- After systemic therapy, choroidal elevation and secondary features of disease resolve, leaving varying degrees of RPE destruction and deposition of hyperreflective subretinal material.

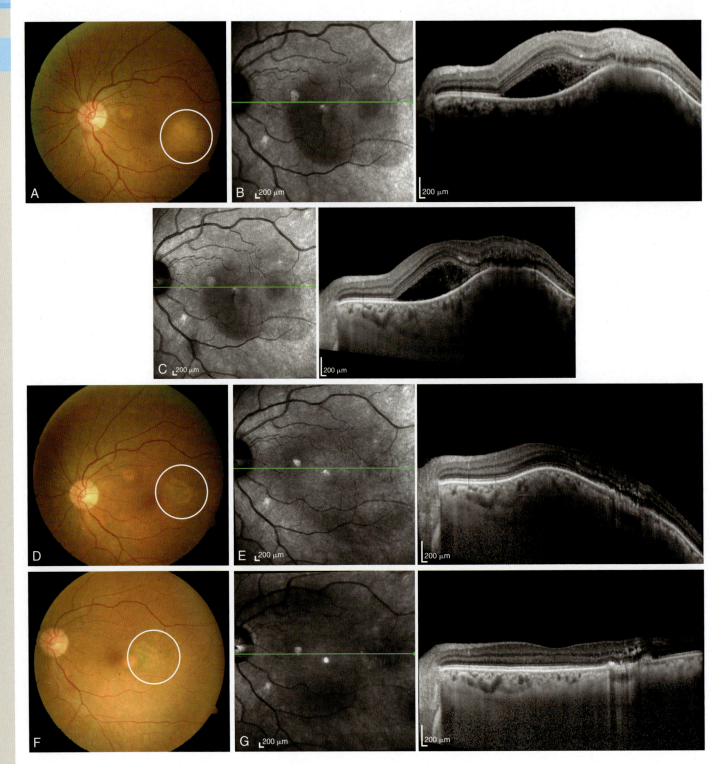

FIG. 19.3.1 (A) Color photograph of choroidal granuloma secondary to tuberculosis *(circle)* before treatment. (B and C) OCT reveals characteristic, dome-shaped, choroidal infiltration. Associated subretinal fluid and subretinal material with mixed reflectivity are present. (D) Color photograph 1 month after systemic therapy. (E) OCT reveals resolution of subretinal fluid and flattening of the choroidal infiltration. (F) Color photograph 3 months after treatment. (G) OCT shows complete resolution of choroidal infiltration, with restoration of a flat retinal pigment epithelium (RPE) contour. Some RPE abnormalities remain temporally. (Courtesy Alay S. Banker, MD.)

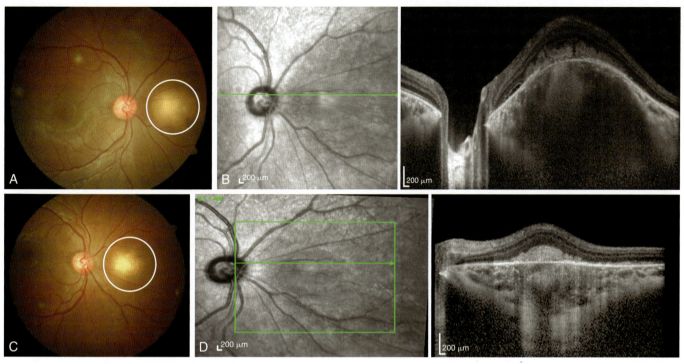

FIG. 19.3.2 (A) Color photograph of choroidal granuloma secondary to tuberculosis. (B) OCT shows significant choroidal infiltration, mild subretinal fluid, and hyperreflective subretinal material. (C) At 4 months after systemic therapy, the choroidal granuloma has become atrophic. (D) OCT shows resolution of choroidal infiltration with flattening of the retinal pigment epithelium. Significant hyperreflective subretinal material remains. (Courtesy Alay S. Banker, MD.)

Posterior Scleritis 19.4

Darin R. Goldman

Summary

The sclera is an opaque structure lining the exterior of the globe that provides structural support and is integral to the function of various ocular structures. Posterior scleritis is the rarest subtype of scleritis, occurring in less than 5% of all cases, defined by inflammation of the posterior sclera. The underlying causes of posterior scleritis are myriad and include both infectious and autoimmune processes, although no cause is identified frequently. The condition may be bilateral, usually with an indolent onset. Pain is a salient feature, and visual acuity may be normal or reduced. The diagnosis of posterior scleritis is difficult to establish because of its low incidence and ability to mimic other pathologic states. Fluorescein angiography, ultrasonography, and orbital radiologic imaging are useful adjunctive diagnostic tests. OCT can provide additional supportive evidence to corroborate the diagnosis while definitively identifying secondary features of posterior scleritis, which may not be obvious by other means. OCT is very sensitive in detecting both chorioretinal folds and serous retinal detachment, both common features of posterior scleritis (Figs. 19.4.1 and 19.4.2). Additionally, OCT provides a particularly useful manner of monitoring therapeutic response to treatment.

Key OCT Features

- Undulations of the retinal pigment epithelium (RPE) in an irregular, wavelike pattern indicate chorioretinal folds, which are common in posterior scleritis.
- Subretinal fluid, often overlying chorioretinal folds, indicates serous retinal detachment. This fluid may be subclinical and thus visible only on OCT.

BIBLIOGRAPHY

Benson, W. E. (1988). Posterior scleritis. *Survey of Ophthalmology 32*(5), 297–316.

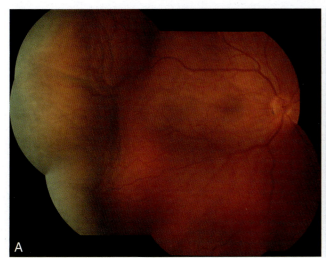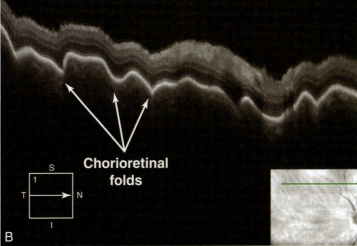

FIG. 19.4.1 (A) Color photograph montage in posterior scleritis showing chorioretinal folds within the macula and temporal periphery. There is a sizable choroidal detachment temporally. (B) OCT on the edge of the superior macula illustrates the typical appearance of chorioretinal folds in posterior scleritis. The retinal pigment epithelium has an irregular, wavelike configuration.

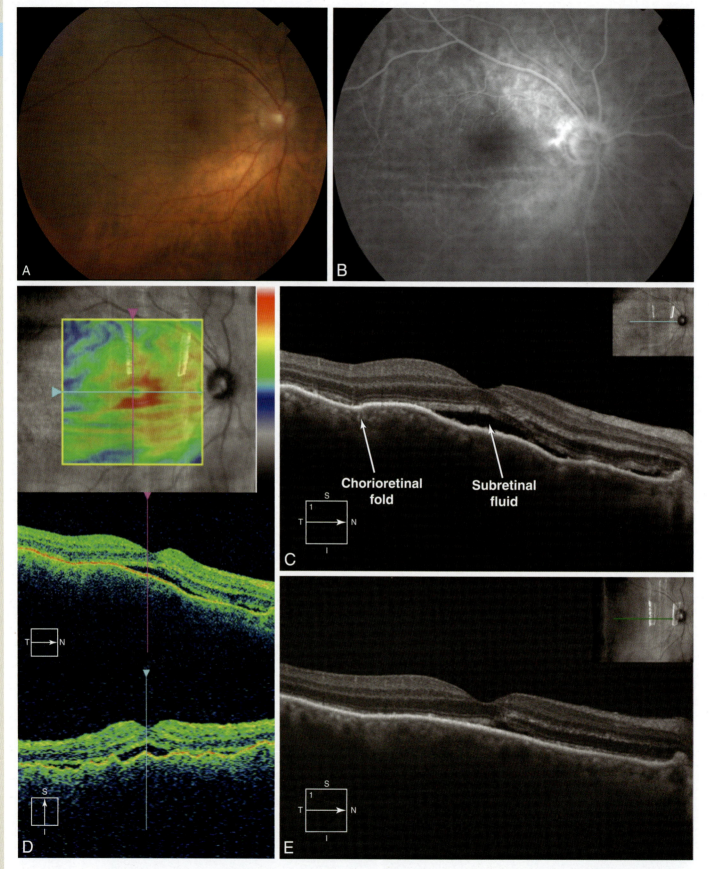

FIG. 19.4.2 (A) Color photograph in posterior scleritis does not illustrate pathologic findings because they are not readily visible clinically. (B) Fluorescein angiography illustrates chorioretinal secondary to alternating stretching and squeezing of the retinal pigment epithelium (RPE) with resultant bands of relative hyper reflectivity and hyporeflectivity. (C) Structural OCT identifies subclinical subretinal fluid and mild chorioretinal folds. (D) Typical appearance of chorioretinal folds on OCT thickness map is shown (*top*). There are bands of varying thickness that result from the undulation of the underlying RPE and subsequent wavelike alteration in the automated inner limiting membrane to RPE thickness that is computed to generate the thickness map. (E) Treatment response to systemic steroids is illustrated with near resolution of chorioretinal folds and subretinal fluid (corresponding to panel C).

Candida Chorioretinitis 19.5

Darin R. Goldman

Summary

Fungal chorioretinitis is a rare ocular disorder that may be acquired via hematogenous dissemination in the setting of fungemia (endogenous) or by direct inoculation in the setting of postoperative infection (exogenous). The most common etiologic pathogen in cases of fungal chorioretinitis are *Candida* species, specifically *Candida albicans*. Although patients with endogenous fungal chorioretinitis are often hospitalized where OCT evaluation is impractical, ambulatory patients also can be affected. Thus, fungal chorioretinitis may be encountered in the outpatient setting, where OCT is readily available. In this setting, diagnosis can be particularly challenging because of limitations in obtaining an adequate specimen and length of time required for confirmatory culture results. OCT is particularly useful to identify characteristic features of fungal chorioretinitis, which can aid in formulating an already challenging diagnosis (Figs. 19.5.1–19.5.3).

Key OCT Features

- Dome-shaped lesion with highly reflective surface and a variable, but significant, degree of underlying shadowing (Fig. 19.5.1B).
- Extensive infection results in diffuse hyperreflective material on the surface of the retina, which may be detectable only on OCT (Fig. 19.5.2B).
- Poor signal strength is common because of media opacity from overlying vitreous involvement.
- Lesions resolve following appropriate antifungal therapy, leaving full-thickness retinal disruption and choroidal atrophy (Fig. 19.5.3D,E).

BIBLIOGRAPHY

Adam, M. K., & Rahimy, E. (2015). Enhanced depth imaging optical coherence tomography of endogenous fungal chorioretinitis. *JAMA Ophthalmology 133*(11), e151931.

Lavine, J. A., & Mititelu, M. (2015). Multimodal imaging of refractory *Candida* chorioretinitis progressing to endogenous endophthalmitis. *Journal of Ophthalmic Inflammation and Infection 5*(1), 54.

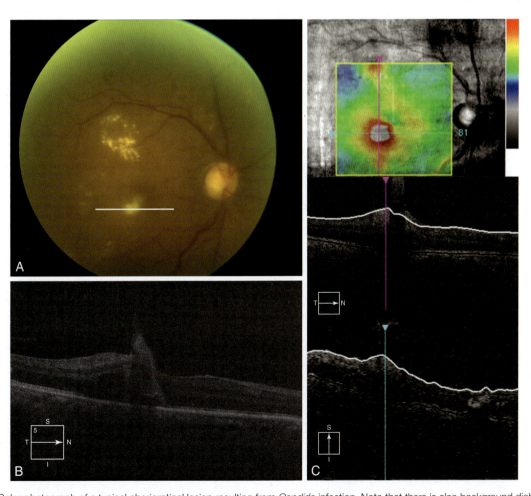

FIG. 19.5.1 (A) Color photograph of a typical chorioretinal lesion resulting from *Candida* infection. Note that there is also background diabetic retinopathy with exudate. (B) OCT through the macular lesion shows full-thickness retinal involvement. (C) OCT thickness map highlights the focal lesion.

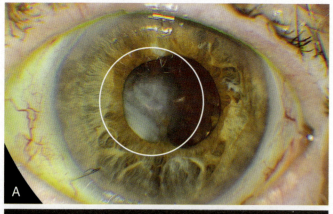

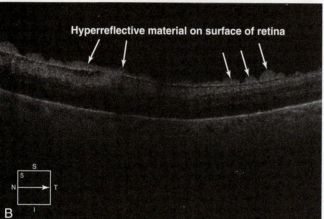

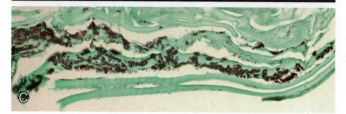

FIG. 19.5.2 (A) Anterior segment photograph of postoperative endophthalmitis caused by *Candida parapsilosis* shows a visible nidus of infected material within the capsular bag *(circle)*. (B) OCT at the edge of the macula shows a sheet of hyperreflective material lining the surface of the retina, which is a feature of extensive infection and was not visible clinically. (C) Grocott-Gomori methenamine silver stain of the lens capsule, which was removed at the time of vitrectomy, shows extensive *Candida parapsilosis* organisms *(dark material)*.

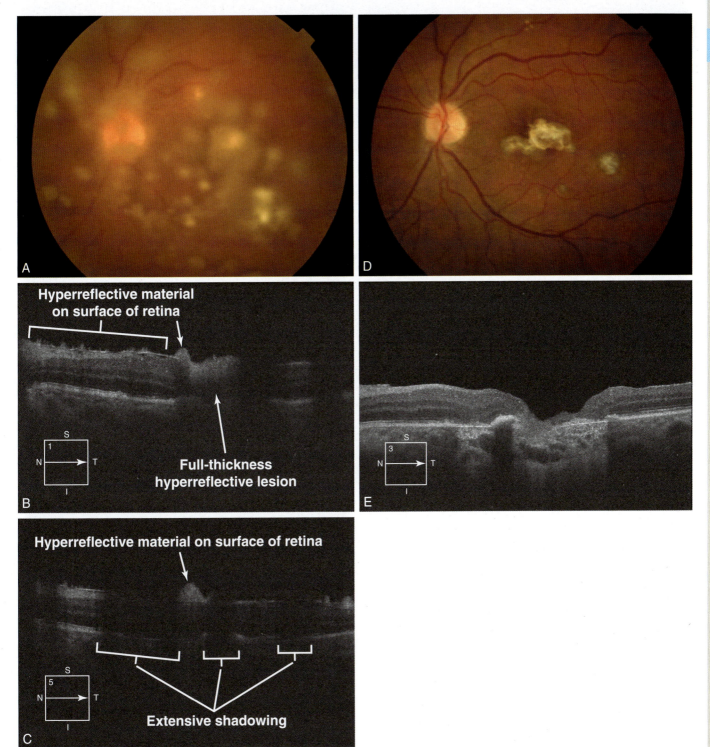

FIG. 19.5.3 (A) Color photograph in a patient with bilateral endogenous endophthalmitis as a result of *Candida albicans*. (B) OCT shows extensive hyperreflective material on the retinal surface and a full-thickness hyperreflective retinal lesion. (C) Extensive shadowing is present because of overlying vitreous involvement, although preretinal hyperreflective lesions are still visible. (D) Chorioretinitis is resolved 6 months following antifungal treatment, leaving extensive chorioretinal atrophy. (E) Corresponding OCT reveals chorioretinal atrophy with varying degrees of retinal layer disorganization. (Courtesy Larry S. Halperin, MD.)

Acute Retinal Necrosis Syndrome | 19.6

Darin R. Goldman

Summary

Acute retinal necrosis syndrome is a severe, vision-threatening viral infection of the retina, most frequently caused by viruses in the herpetic family. The retinal necrosis typically begins in the peripheral retina in a sporadic array of opaque, white patches that are well circumscribed. These patches rapidly coalesce in a circumferential trajectory, becoming confluent over time and spreading posteriorly. Associated retinal occlusive vasculitis and uveitis are common features. Choroiditis and subclinical serous retinal detachment also may be present, which can be identified using OCT. In the acute setting, clinically evident, full-thickness retinal whitening appears on OCT as diffuse, homogeneous hyperreflectivity with variable thickening of the retina (Fig. 19.6.1). The inner retina may become involved initially, followed by rapid involvement of the entire thickness of the retina. Within days to weeks, the retinal layers become disorganized and generalized atrophy appears. The remaining retinal tissue maintains a diffusely hyperreflective signal. Over time, complete loss of retinal layers may develop, leaving hyporeflective cavities. Secondary retinal detachment is a common late complication. Although OCT findings in acute retinal necrosis syndrome are not specific, they serve as a useful adjunct in the diagnostic evaluation.

Key OCT Features

- In the acute phase of acute retinal necrosis syndrome, there is full-thickness, diffuse hyperreflectivity of the retina in a well-defined area, corresponding to clinically evident retinal necrosis.
- Subclinical overlying vitreous inflammation, subretinal fluid, or choroidal thickening may be visible on OCT.
- Over time, retinal thinning and loss of tissue often develop in areas of prior retinal necrosis, despite antiviral therapy.

BIBLIOGRAPHY

Duker, J. S., & Blumenkranz, M. S. (1991). Diagnosis and management of the acute retinal necrosis (ARN) syndrome. *Survey of Ophthalmology*, 35, 327–343.

Kurup, S. P., Khan, S., & Gill, M. K. (2014). Spectral domain optical coherence tomography in the evaluation and management of infectious retinitis. *Retina*, 34(11), 2233–2241.

Murata, K., Yamada, W., Nishida, T., Murase, H., Ishida, K., Mochizuki, K., et al. (2016). Sequential optical coherence tomography images of early macular necrosis caused by acute retinal necrosis in non-human immunodeficiency virus patients. *Retina*, 36(7), e55–e57.

Ohtake-Matsumoto, A., Keino, H., Koto, T., & Okada, A. A. (2015). Spectral domain and swept source optical coherence tomography findings in acute retinal necrosis. *Graefe's Archive for Clinical and Experimental Ophthalmology*, 253(11), 2049–2051.

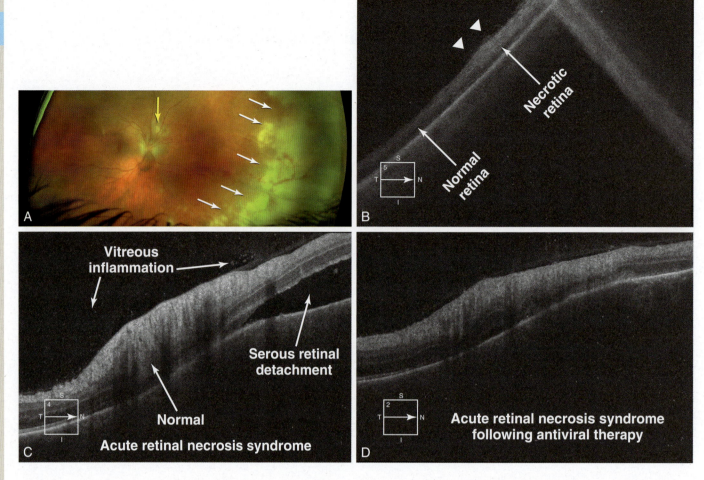

FIG. 19.6.1 (A) Wide-angle image of acute retinal necrosis syndrome involving the nasal periphery *(white arrows)*. A satellite lesion is also present above the optic nerve *(yellow arrow)*. (B) The nasal periphery is imaged at the transition from normal to necrotic retina. The necrotic retina is diffusely hyperreflective with mild thickening and overlying vitreous inflammation *(arrowheads)*. (C) The satellite lesion above the optic nerve is imaged in cross-section. There is diffuse hyperreflectivity throughout the involved region of the retina with significant thickening. Associated subclinical serous retinal detachment, choroidal enlargement, and vitreous inflammation are also present. (D) Same section as in part C 2 weeks after antiviral therapy shows less retinal hyperreflectivity, vitreous inflammation, and choroidal thickening along with resolution of subretinal fluid. (Courtesy Eduardo Uchiyama, MD.)

Choroidal Nevus

Angell Shi | Shilpa J. Desai*

20.1

Summary

Choroidal nevi are common, benign, typically flat, variably pigmented lesions of the choroid. Nevi do not usually grow but can become increasingly pigmented, acquire drusen on the surface, and be associated with subretinal fluid, which is often detectable only on OCT. Photoreceptor loss or attenuation may or may not be present. In most cases, increased thickness of the retinal pigment epithelium (RPE)/choriocapillaris layer and hyporeflectivity within the anterior portion of the nevus can be seen, particularly in those that are pigmented. Nevi can transform into melanoma, although this is quite rare. Risk factors for malignant transformation include thickness over 2 mm, presence of subretinal fluid, symptoms such as vision loss, orange pigment (due to surface lipofuscin), juxtapapillary location, lack of overlying drusen, and hollowness on ultrasonography. Clinically, choroidal nevi appear as darkly pigmented, round lesions located beneath the retina (Fig. 20.1.1). Typical size ranges from 1 to 4 disc diameters, although larger nevi may occur. Choroidal nevi may be located throughout the fundus. Clinical photographs are the best method of documenting their appearance. OCT provides adjunctive information and may help confirm the diagnosis in uncertain cases.

Key OCT Features

- Flat to minimal thickening is seen.
- Well-defined blocking of signal occurs in the outer choroid.
- Overlying choriocapillaris is compressed (Fig. 20.1.2).
- Overlying retina may have cystic changes or localized subretinal fluid.

BIBLIOGRAPHY

Chien, J. L., Sofi, K., Surakiatchanukul, T., Shields, J. A., & Shields, C. L. (2017). Choroidal nevus: A review of prevalence, features, genetics, risks, and outcomes. *Current Opinion in Ophthalmology, 28*(3), 228–237.

Say, E. A., Shah, S. U., Ferenczy, S., & Shields, C. L. (2012). Optical coherence tomography of retinal and choroidal tumors. *Journal of Ophthalmology, 2012*, 385058.

Shields, C. L., Furuta, M., Mashayekhi, A., Berman, E. L., Zahler, J. D., Hoberman, D. M., et al. (2008). Clinical spectrum of choroidal nevi based on age at presentation in 3422 consecutive eyes. *Ophthalmology, 115*(3), 546–552.e2.

FIG. 20.1.1 Fundus photograph of a 3 × 2-mm nonsuspicious choroidal nevus.

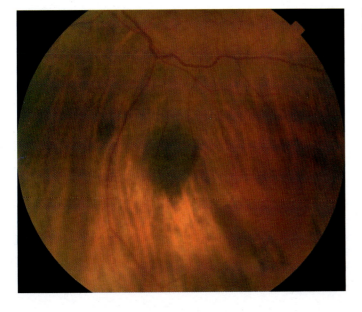

*With contributions from Jay S. Duker

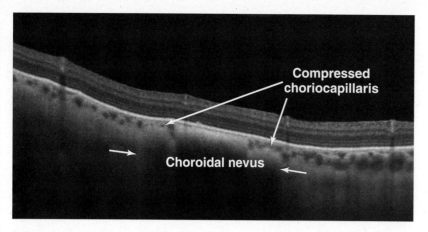

FIG. 20.1.2 Spectral domain OCT line scan through a 3 × 2-mm nonsuspicious choroidal nevus. Note intact overlying retina and no subretinal fluid. There is compression of the choriocapillaris. The nevus itself is located in the outer choroid and blocks penetration of the OCT signal.

Choroidal Melanoma | 20.2

Angell Shi | Shilpa J. Desai*

Summary

Choroidal melanoma is the most common primary malignancy of the posterior segment of the eye in adults. In nearly every instance, they occur unilaterally and unifocally. They are usually pigmented, typically tan to dark brown in color, but may be completely amelanotic. While most are dome or mushroom shaped, diffuse melanoma is relatively flat and can be mistaken for a nevus. Choroidal melanomas vary in size (both in diameter and in thickness), although larger and more elevated lesions are more likely to be melanoma in comparison to nevi and tend to be associated with a worse prognosis. When they metastasize, the liver is the primary site of hematogenous spread. B-scan ultrasonography is an adjunctive imaging modality that may be helpful for measuring and monitoring tumor dimensions. Histologic and cytogenetic studies can provide further classification and prognostication.

Key OCT Features

- Elevated choroidal mass with extensive blocking of signal (Fig. 20.2.1).
- Overlying subretinal fluid is present with shaggy photoreceptors (Fig. 20.2.1).
- Obscuration of the normal choroidal vascular pattern in the area of the tumor (Fig. 20.2.2).

BIBLIOGRAPHY

Shields, C. L., Kaliki, S., Furuta, M., Mashayekhi, A., & Shields, J. A. (2012). Clinical spectrum and prognosis of uveal melanoma based on age at presentation in 8,033 cases. *Retina, 32*(7), 1363–1372.

Say, E. A., Shah, S. U., Ferenczy, S., & Shields, C. L. (2012). Optical coherence tomography of retinal and choroidal tumors. *Journal of Ophthalmology, 2012*, 385058.

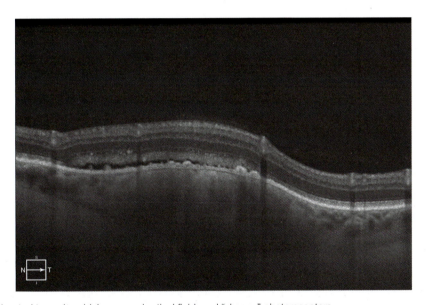

FIG. 20.2.1 OCT showing elevated transchoroidal mass, subretinal fluid, and "shaggy" photoreceptors.

*With contributions from Jay S. Duker

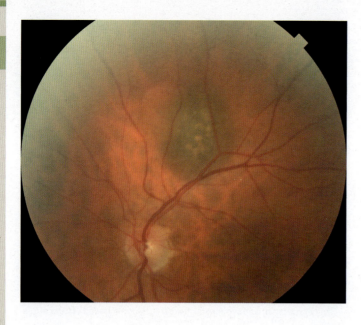

FIG. 20.2.2 Color figure corresponding to OCT in Fig. 20.2.1 showing a small choroidal melanoma measuring 7 mm in diameter and 2 mm in thickness.

Solitary Choroidal Hemangioma

Yi Ling Dai | Shilpa J. Desai*

20.3

Summary

Solitary choroidal hemangioma is a benign lesion of the choroid that typically presents in the fourth or fifth decade of life (Shields et al., 2001). These lesions become apparent when leakage into the retina or subretinal space results in symptoms or they are identified during routine ophthalmologic examination. The lesions are typically round or oval in shape, red in coloration, and between 3 and 4 mm in thickness (Fig. 20.3.1). Overlying cystic retinal degeneration, subretinal fluid, and retinal pigment epithelial changes are common (Karimi et al., 2015; Shields et al., 2001). Treatment is indicated only if central acuity is affected. Laser photocoagulation, photodynamic therapy, and low-dose radiation can be successful in eliminating the fluid leakage (Di Nicola et al., 2020; Karimi et al., 2015; Shields et al., 2001).

Key OCT Findings

- Localized choroidal mass with large inherent vasculature.
- Subretinal fluid and cystic retinal degeneration may be present over the tumor.
- Tumor mass exhibits a hyporeflective internal signal (Fig. 20.3.2).

REFERENCES

Di Nicola, M., Williams, B. K., Jr., Srinivasan, A., Al-Dahmash, S., Mashayekhi, A., Shields, J. A., et al. (2020). Photodynamic therapy for circumscribed choroidal hemangioma in 79 consecutive patients: Comparative analysis of factors predictive of visual outcome. *Ophthalmology. Retina*, 4(10), 1024–1033. https://doi.org/10.1016/j.oret.2020.04.018.

Karimi, S., Nourinia, R., & Mashayekhi, A. (2015). Circumscribed choroidal hemangioma. *Journal of Ophthalmic & Vision Research*, 10(3), 320–328. https://doi.org/10.4103/2008-322X.170353.

Shields, C. L., Honavar, S. G., Shields, J. A., Cater, J., & Demirci, H. (2001). Circumscribed choroidal hemangioma: clinical manifestations and factors predictive of visual outcome in 200 consecutive cases [published correction appears in *Ophthalmology* 2002 Feb;109(2):222]. *Ophthalmology*, 108(12), 2237–2248. https://doi.org/10.1016/s0161-6420(01)00812-0.

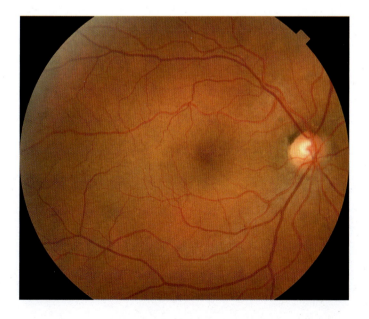

FIG. 20.3.1 Color fundus photograph showing subtle reddish mass superior to disc.

---

*With contributions from Jay S. Duker

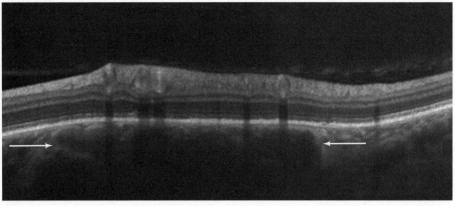

FIG. 20.3.2 OCT of solitary choroidal hemangioma, which is located between the two *arrows*. Note the generalized hyporeflectivity of the lesion.

Retinal Capillary Hemangioma | 21.1

Yi Ling Dai | Shilpa J. Desai*

Summary

Retinal capillary hemangiomas, also known as retinal capillary hemangioblastomas or retinal angiomas, are benign lesions that can develop either as an isolated phenomenon or in association with Von-Hippel Lindau syndrome (Gass & Braunstein, 1980; Maher et al., 1990). The lesions are round or oval and typically have enlarged, dilated feeding and draining retinal vessels (Colvard et al., 1978). Early in their course, hemangiomas rarely cause visual issues, but over time, they can grow and cause both intraretinal and subretinal fluid accumulation with hard exudate, both locally around the tumor and at a distance in the macula. Over time, vitreous traction can develop with resultant retinal detachment (Maher et al., 1990). Treatment may vary from observation to plaque therapy, depending on the location, tumor size, and degree of visual involvement (Singh et al., 2002).

Key OCT Features

- Secondary macular edema, hard exudate, and subretinal fluid due to leaking peripheral retinal capillary hemangiomas can be identified (Figs. 21.1.1–21.1.3).
- Vitreous changes over capillary hemangiomas are common.
- The lesions are elevated and well circumscribed but show little internal detail.

REFERENCES

Colvard, D. M., Robertson, D. M., & Traytmann, J. C. (1978). Cavernous hemangioma of the retina. *Archives of Ophthalmology*, 96, 2042–2044.

Gass, J. D., & Braunstein, R. (1980). Sessile and exophytic capillary angiomas of the juxtapapillary retina and optic nerve head. *Archives of Ophthalmology*, 98, 1790–1797.

Maher, E. R., Yates, J. R., Harries, R., Benjamin, C., Harris, R., Moore, A. T., et al. (1990). Clinical features and natural history of von Hippel Lindau disease. *The Quarterly Journal of Medicine*, 77, 1151–1163.

Singh, A. D., Nouri, M., Shields, C. L., Shields, J. A., & Perez, N. (2002). Treatment of retinal capillary hemangioma. *Ophthalmology*, 109(10), 1799–1806. https://doi.org/10.1016/s0161-6420(02)01177-6.

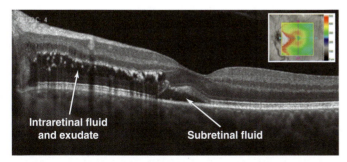

FIG. 21.1.1 Macular OCT in a patient with a peripheral retinal capillary hemangioma. Intraretinal fluid, subretinal fluid, and exudate are all common features that may be present.

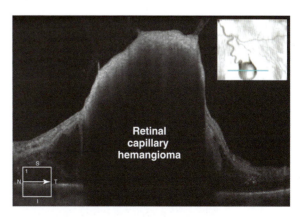

FIG. 21.1.2 Peripheral OCT in the same patient as in Fig. 21.1.1 through the center of the retinal capillary hemangioma. The surface of the lesion is hyperreflective, and the vitreoretinal interface exhibits sites of adhesion. Internal details are not visualized because of significant shadowing of the signal.

*With contributions from Jay S. Duker

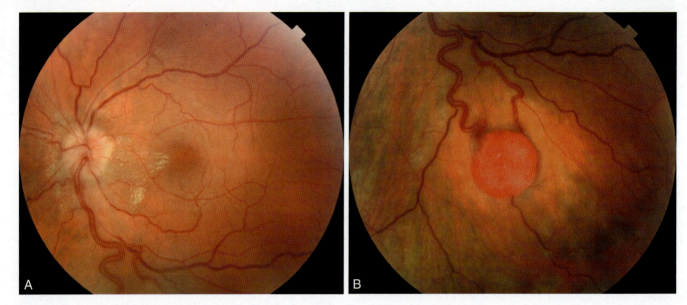

FIG. 21.1.3 (A) Color photographs of the macula (corresponding to Fig. 21.1.1) and (B) the peripheral lesion (corresponding to Fig. 21.1.2).

Simple Hamartoma of the RPE

Erin M. Lanzo | Shilpa J. Desai*

22.1

Summary

Congenital simple hamartoma of the retinal pigment epithelium (RPE) is an uncommon, benign tumor of the RPE that appears as a jet-black, well-demarcated, round lesion on the foveal surface. The location on the retinal surface may be explained by aberrant migration during embryogenesis. Although the lesions are thought to be congenital, they are typically an incidental finding identified during routine ophthalmoscopy in asymptomatic adults. The clinical appearance is suggestive, and the OCT appearance is pathognomonic of the diagnosis. Observation is generally recommended in the absence of visual symptoms, although decreased acuity due to secondary epiretinal membrane formation and foveal vitreomacular traction has been described (Barnes et al., 2014).

Key OCT Features

- Preretinal location with dense hyperreflectivity that results in shadowing and obscuration of both the underlying retina and choriocapillaris (Figs. 22.1.1 and 22.1.2).
- Extremely sharply demarcated borders.

REFERENCE

Barnes, A. C., Goldman, D. R., Laver, N. V., & Duker, J. S. (2014). Congenital simple hamartoma of the retinal pigment epithelium: Clinical, optical coherence tomography, and histopathological correlation. *Eye (London), 28*(6), 765–766.

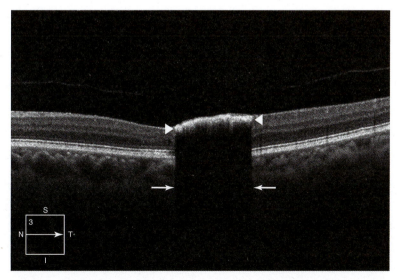

FIG. 22.1.1 OCT of typical simple hamartoma of the retinal pigment epithelium. The lesion is located between the *arrowheads* and exhibits extreme hyperreflectivity. The extent of the underlying shadowing is shown between the *arrows*.

---

*With contributions from Jay S. Duker

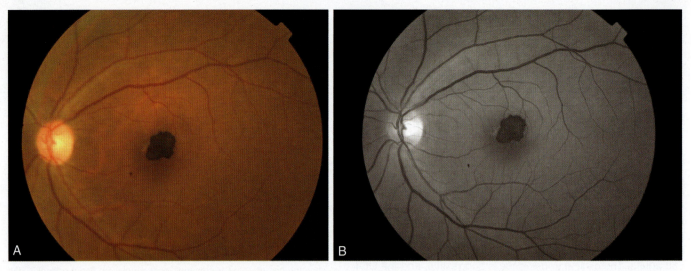

FIG. 22.1.2 Color (A) and red-free (B) photographs (corresponding to Fig. 22.1.1) illustrate the jet-black color and typical clinical appearance of congenital simple hamartoma of the retinal pigment epithelium.

Combined Hamartoma of the Retina and RPE | 22.2

Tavish Nanda | Shilpa J. Desai*

Summary

Combined hamartoma of the retina and retinal pigment epithelium (RPE) is a rare, benign hamartomatous growth. It is important to distinguish this entity from others that may appear similar, but are malignant, such as adenocarcinoma of the RPE and retinoblastoma. The usual clinical appearance is a peripapillary, pigmented, focal disorganization of the retina, with overlying fibrosis. The involved region includes full-thickness retina and RPE. The central macula can be disrupted by secondary vitreoretinal interface forces or by the lesion itself, resulting in visual impairment. OCT is extremely useful in confirming the diagnosis and examining the affected tissues. In particular, there is often inner retinal contracture, an overlying epiretinal membrane, and an absence of choroidal involvement.

Key OCT Features

- Full-thickness retinal and RPE disorganization is present in most cases (Fig. 22.2.1).
- Overlying fibrosis is present, often with a sawtooth pattern (Figs. 22.2.1 and 22.2.2).
- Cystoid macular edema, epiretinal membrane, and tractional retinal detachment may be present as secondary features (Fig. 22.2.1).

BIBLIOGRAPHY

Shields, C. L., Mashayekhi, A., Dai, V. V., Materin, M. A., & Shields, J. A. (2005). Optical coherence tomographic findings of combined hamartoma of the retina and retinal pigment epithelium in 11 patients. *Archives of Ophthalmology, 123*(12), 1746–1750.

Xue, K., Mellington, F., Gout, I., Rokerya, S., Ibironke Olurin, O., & El-Amir, A. (2012). Combined hamartoma of the retina and retinal pigment epithelium. *BMJ Case Reports 2012*, bcr2012006944 https://doi.org/10.1136/bcr-2012-006944.

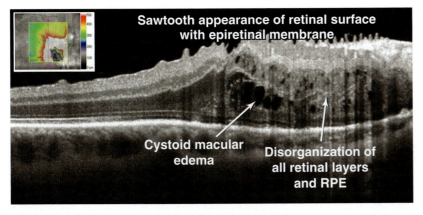

Sawtooth appearance of retinal surface with epiretinal membrane

Cystoid macular edema

Disorganization of all retinal layers and RPE

FIG. 22.2.1 OCT appearance of a typical combined hamartoma of the retina and RPE. *RPE*, Retinal pigment epithelium.

*With contributions from Jay S. Duker

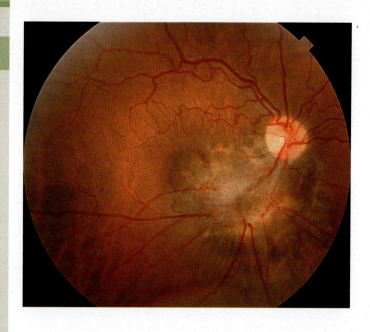

FIG. 22.2.2 Corresponding color photograph to Fig. 22.2.1.

Choroidal Metastases

Erin M. Lanzo | Shilpa J. Desai*

23.1

Summary

Choroidal metastases are rare but represent the most common malignancy of the posterior segment in adults. The most common sites of primary lesions are the breast and lung. Metastases are often multiple and bilateral (Arepalli et al., 2015). Treatment in the form of systemic chemotherapy, immunotherapy, hormone therapy, or whole eye radiotherapy is recommended for active, multifocal, or bilateral lesions. Plaque radiotherapy, transpupillary radiotherapy, or photodynamic therapy may be considered for active solitary metastases. Radiation is often successful at halting growth of the lesions, but the systemic prognosis in most cases is poor.

Key OCT Features

- Dense choroidal mass with little to no visible choroidal vasculature (Figs. 23.1.1 and 23.1.2).
- Retinal pigment epithelium tends to assume a "wavelike," "lumpy-bumpy," or irregular lobulated configuration with underlying choroidal thickening.
- Overlying subretinal fluid is very common (Witkin et al., 2012).

REFERENCES

Arepalli, S., Kaliki, S., & Shields, C. L. (2015). Choroidal metastases: Origin, features, and therapy. *Indian Journal of Ophthalmology*, 63(2), 122–127.

Witkin, A. J., Fischer, D. H., Shields, C. L., Reichstein, D., & Shields, J. A. (2012). Enhanced depth imaging spectral-domain optical coherence tomography of a subtle choroidal metastasis. *Eye*, 26, 1598–1599.

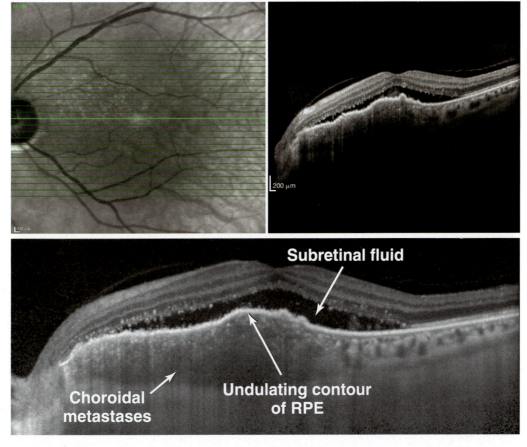

FIG. 23.1.1 OCT of choroidal metastasis exhibits characteristic infiltration of the choriocapillaris, undulating contour of the RPE, and overlying subretinal fluid. *RPE,* Retinal pigment epithelium.

*With contributions from Jay S. Duker

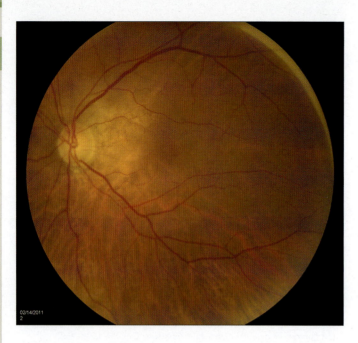

FIG. 23.1.2 Corresponding color fundus photograph shows the amelanotic choroidal mass just temporal to the optic nerve.

Valsalva Retinopathy

Allison Resnik | Shilpa J. Desai*

24.1

Summary

Valsalva retinopathy is caused by the rupture of superficial capillaries within the inner retina. Inciting events include anything in which forced exhalation against a closed glottis occurs, which results in a sudden increase in intraocular venous pressure. Resultant hemorrhage pools within the sub–inner limiting membrane (ILM) space, typically overlying the macula. The acute hemorrhage becomes layered with time because of gravitational dependence, resulting in the characteristic "double ring sign." Over time, most cases resolve spontaneously. OCT is useful in identifying the location of the hemorrhage within the sub-ILM space and confirms the diagnosis in the appropriate clinical context. Additionally, OCT provides a precise modality for monitoring the hemorrhage size and volume.

Key OCT Features

- Vertically oriented OCT scanning patterns are most useful.
- On vertical OCT, two distinct areas are present within the sub-ILM space (Fig. 24.1.1):
  1. Superior hyporeflective cavity (serous component)
  2. Inferior hyperreflective cavity (hemorrhagic component)
- Comparing registered vertical OCT scans or volume cube scans over time can definitively determine the clinical course (Figs. 24.1.1 and 24.1.2).

BIBLIOGRAPHY

Goldman, D. R., & Baumal, C. R. (2014). Natural history of Valsalva retinopathy in an adolescent. *Journal of Pediatric Ophthalmology and Strabismus*, *51*(2), 128.

Szelog, J. T., Lally, D. R., & Heier, J. S. (2015). Natural history of Valsalva-induced subhyaloid hemorrhage. *JAMA Ophthalmology*, *133*(2), e143268.

---

*With contributions from Jay S. Duker

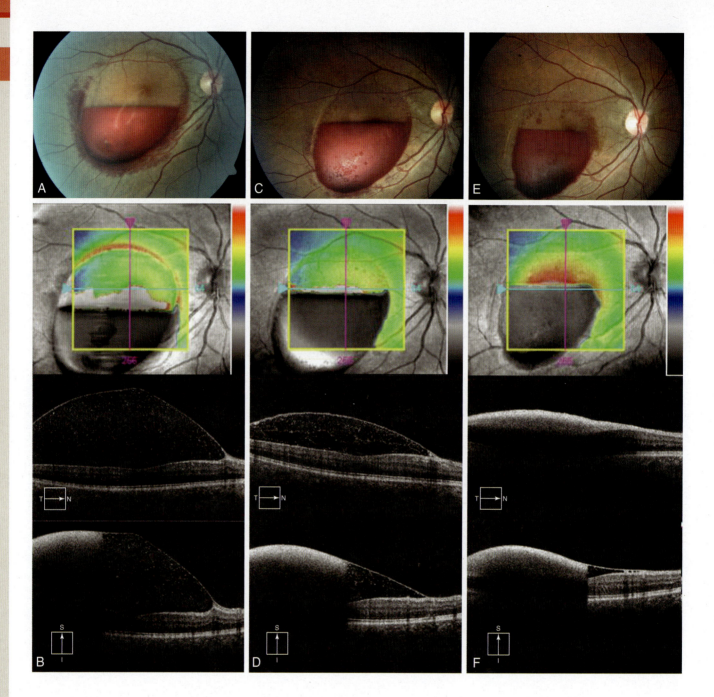

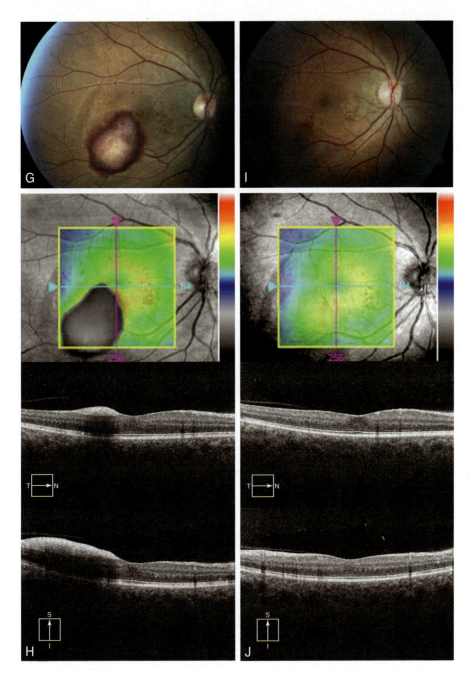

FIG. 24.1.1 A 33-year-old healthy woman with Valsalva retinopathy secondary to vigorous vomiting related to cholecystitis. (A and B) At 1 week after symptom onset, there is layered hemorrhage in the sub–inner limiting membrane space. Visual acuity measured 20/200. (C and D) At 2 weeks after presentation, visual acuity measured 20/200, and the vertical height of the hemorrhage clinically appears to have increased compared to that at presentation. However, the OCT confirms that the total hemorrhage volume has actually contracted significantly. (E and F) At 1 month after presentation, visual acuity measured 20/100, with continued contracture of the hemorrhage. (G and H) At 2 months after presentation, visual acuity improved to 20/25, with clearance of the hemorrhage from the central fovea. (I and J) At 4 months after presentation, visual acuity returned to 20/20, with complete resolution of hemorrhage.

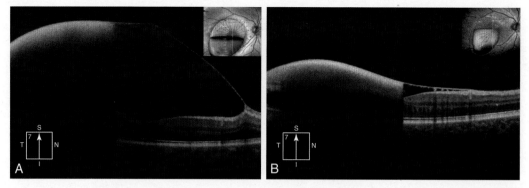

FIG. 24.1.2 Comparison of sub–inner limiting membrane hemorrhage in Valsalva retinopathy as seen on vertically oriented OCT scans at baseline (A) and 1 month after presentation (B).

Laser Maculopathy

Allison Resnik | Shilpa J. Desai*

25.1

Summary

High-powered lasers have become common in both the commercial and recreational setting, given the ease in accessibility and lack of regulation from online retailers. This provides an opportunity for both accidental and purposeful laser exposure to the macula. The central macula generally receives most of the injury due to the direct visualization of the laser beam. Clinically, the acute lesion appears yellow and mottled and fades quickly over weeks to months. The later stages of injury are nonspecific, with varying amounts of retinal pigment epithelium (RPE) pigmentary disturbances and retinal atrophy. The extent of retinal injury depends on the burden of exposure, with mild injuries affecting only the outer retina; more severe injuries can affect the full retinal thickness.

Key OCT Features

- In the acute setting, there is localized outer > inner retinal involvement, with curvilinear hyperreflective bands involving the inner segment/outer segment/ellipsoid zone (IS/OS/EZ) and RPE (Figs. 25.1.1 and 25.1.2).
- In the subacute or chronic setting, patchy RPE disruption and clumping are present (Fig. 25.1.3).
- IS/OS/EZ normalization varies depending on severity of initial injury (i.e., wavelength, power, and duration of exposure of laser device) and correlates with visual recovery.

BIBLIOGRAPHY

Bhavsar, K. V., Wilson, D., Margolis, R., Judson, P., Barbazetto, I., Freund, K. B., et al. (2015). Multimodal imaging in handheld laser-induced maculopathy. *American Journal of Ophthalmology*, 159, 227–231.e2.

Wyrsch, S., Baenninger, P. B., & Schmid, M. K. (2010). Retinal injuries from a handheld laser pointer. *New England Journal of Medicine*, 363(11), 1089–1091.

FIG. 25.1.1 OCT of severe acute laser maculopathy.

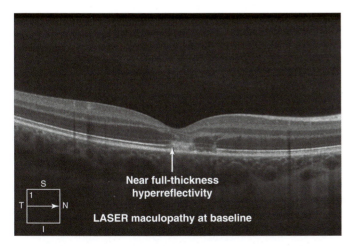

*With contributions from Jay S. Duker

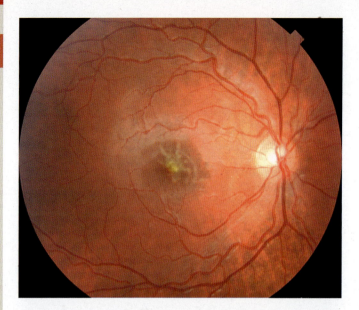

FIG. 25.1.2 Corresponding color photograph to Fig. 25.1.1.

FIG. 25.1.3 OCT 6 weeks after the original injury. *IS/OS/EZ*, Inner segment/outer segment/ellipsoid zone; *RPE*, retinal pigment epithelium.

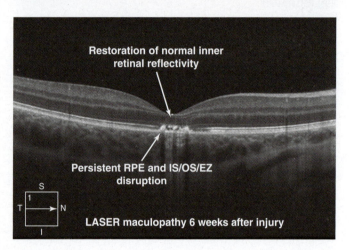

Restoration of normal inner retinal reflectivity

Persistent RPE and IS/OS/EZ disruption

LASER maculopathy 6 weeks after injury

Solar Maculopathy

Chelsea Gottschalk | Shilpa J. Desai

25.2

Summary

Accidental or purposeful prolonged exposure to intense light sources such as the sun (as may happen in psychiatric disease or during a solar eclipse), a welding arc, or an operating microscope can result in photochemical injury to the macula. The injury is typically bilateral, symmetric, and located within the fovea, although in cases associated with operating microscopes, the lesion is usually inferior to the fovea. Loss of vision occurs as a central scotoma that correlates with the severity of the exposure. OCT findings can be diagnostic in the appropriate clinical context. Initial hyperreflectivity followed by focal outer retinal "holes" in the central fovea are the key finding, which can occasionally be seen in other conditions. There are no treatments available; however, visual prognosis remains good.

Key OCT Features

- The inner retina is normal.
- Focal disruption or loss of the retinal pigment epithelial (RPE) and inner segment/outer segment/ellipsoid zone (IS/IO/EZ), with sharply demarcated borders of normal retina on the edges (Figs. 25.2.1–25.2.3).
- OCT findings are generally present long-term after the initial photic exposure.

BIBLIOGRAPHY

Chen, R. W., Gorczynska, I., Srinivasan, V. J., Fujimoto, J. G., Duker, J. S., & Reichel, E. (2008). High-speed ultrahigh resolution optical coherence tomography findings in chronic solar retinopathy. *Retin Cases Brief Rep, 2*(2), 103–105.

Comander, J., Gardiner, M., & Loewenstein, J. (2011). High-resolution optical coherence tomography findings in solar maculopathy and the differential diagnosis of outer retinal holes. *American Journal of Ophthalmology, 152*(3), 413–419.

Kleinmann, G., Hoffman, P., Schechtman, E., & Pollack, A. (2002). Microscope-induced retinal phototoxicity in cataract surgery of short duration. *American Journal of Ophthalmology, 109*(2), 334–338.

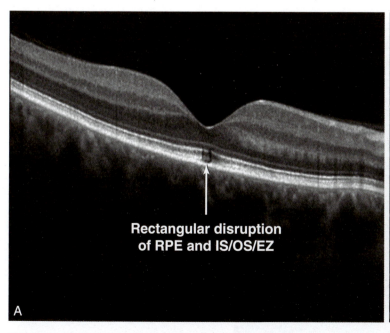
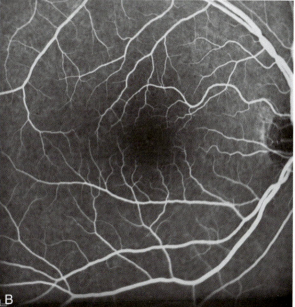

Rectangular disruption of RPE and IS/OS/EZ

FIG. 25.2.1 (A) OCT of solar maculopathy. (B) Corresponding fluorescein angiogram shows pinpoint area of hyperfluorescence. *IS/IO/EZ*, Inner segment/outer segment/ellipsoid zone; *RPE*, Retinal pigment epithelial.

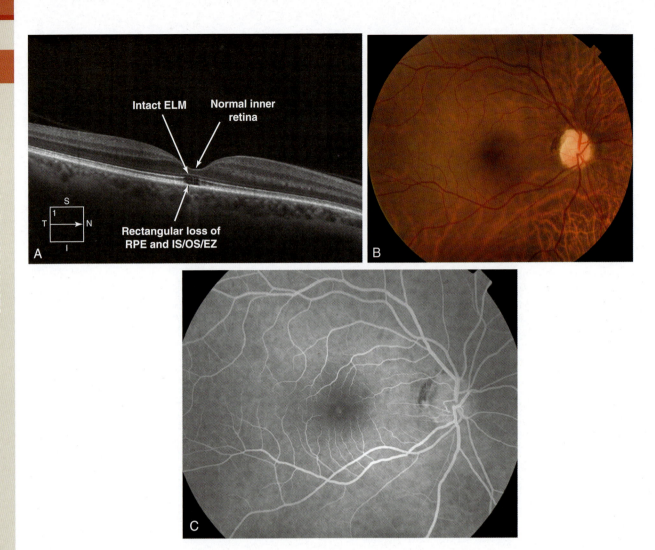

FIG. 25.2.2. Typical appearance of solar maculopathy. (A) OCT. (B) Fundus photograph. (C) Fluorescein angiogram. *ELM*, External limiting membrane; *IS/IO/EZ*, inner segment/outer segment/ellipsoid zone; *RPE*, Retinal pigment epithelial.

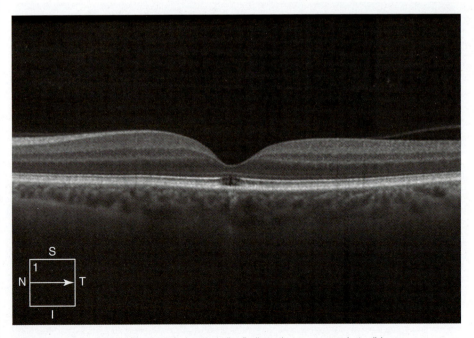

FIG. 25.2.3. Fellow eye of Fig. 25.2.2 shows similar findings that are somewhat milder.

Retinitis Pigmentosa | 26.1

Shilpa J. Desai | A. Yasin Alibhai

Summary

Retinitis pigmentosa (RP) refers to a heterogeneous group of inherited disorders that are characterized by loss of retinal cell function, preferentially in the peripheral retina. RP can have varying severity, age of onset, mode of inheritance, and systemic associations. RP may be inherited in an autosomal dominant, autosomal recessive, or X-linked recessive fashion. The X-linked form of the disease is typically the most severe. The disease is often secondary to mutations in the rhodopsin gene, although some forms have been linked to mutations in the *RDS* gene (Anasagasti et al., 2012). Generally, RP is characterized by a slowly progressive loss of night vision (nyctalopia) along with contraction of the visual field. In later stages of the disease, central acuity is affected, which may cause profound vision loss. Typical fundus abnormalities include waxy pallor of the optic nerve, a tapetal-like reflex resulting from changes in the retinal pigment epithelium (RPE), narrowing of the peripheral retinal vasculature, and bone-spicule changes in the mid-peripheral retina (Fig. 26.1.1). Definitive diagnosis requires electrophysiologic testing. Computed tomography is useful to aid in the initial diagnosis and detecting associated macular abnormalities such as cystoid macular edema (Fig. 26.1.2). Treatment of RP is limited at this time, although retinal prosthetic implants are available for extremely severe cases (Farrar et al., 2012).

Key Features

- Symptoms include nyctalopia, constricted visual field, and, in some cases, profound vision loss.
- Waxy pallor of the optic nerve, attenuation of the retinal vessels, and bone spicules in the peripheral retina are common clinical findings.
- OCT findings in early/milder disease include relative preservation of the central retina and RPE with loss of the outer retina and RPE adjacent to the fovea.
- OCT findings in advanced/severe disease include marked attenuation of all retinal layers, particularly the outer retina and photoreceptors.
- Associated cystoid macular edema may be identified on OCT.

REFERENCES

Anasagasti, A., Irigoyen, C., Barandika, O., López de Munain, A., & Ruiz-Ederra, J. (2012). Current mutation discovery approaches in retinitis pigmentosa. *Vision Research*, *75*, 117–129.

Farrar, G. J., Millington-Ward, S., Chadderton, N., Humphries, P., & Kenna, P. F. (2012). Gene-based therapies for dominantly inherited retinopathies. *Gene Therapy*, *19*(2), 137–144.

BIBLIOGRAPHY

Wolfensberger, T. J. (1999). The role of carbonic anhydrase inhibitors in the management of macular edema. *Documenta Ophthalmologica*, *97*(3–4), 387–397.

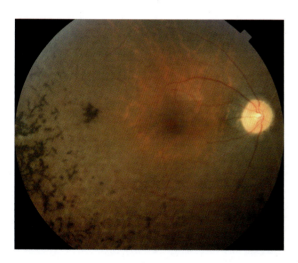

FIG. 26.1.1 Color fundus photograph of a patient with typical retinitis pigmentosa. There is peripheral bone-spicule deposition encroaching into the macula, optic nerve pallor, and prominent vascular attenuation. The central retina and RPE are preserved ("central island").

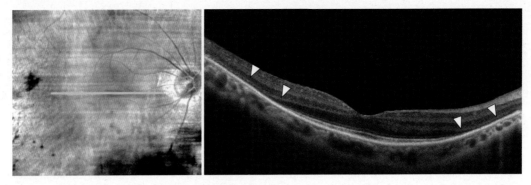

FIG. 26.1.2 OCT B-scan corresponding to Fig. 26.1.1. There is significant thinning of the outer retinal layers and dropout of the RPE involving the edges of the macula. However, the central fovea is spared with normal retinal architecture.

Stargardt Disease | 26.2

Chelsea Gottschalk | Shilpa J. Desai

Summary

Stargardt disease is the most common inheritable macular dystrophy, associated with mutations in the *ABCA4* gene, which accounts for the majority of macular degeneration in young people. The age of onset and disease severity vary, but generally, the longer the duration of disease, the more severe it is. The fundus appearance is that of fleck-like deposits of yellowish material at the level of the retinal pigment epithelium (RPE) in a pattern centered on the macula, although the entire posterior pole may be involved (Fig. 26.2.1). Associated central macular atrophy accounts for vision loss that correlates with its proximity to the foveal center. Fluorescein angiography displays a characteristic dark choroid in the majority of cases due to lipofuscin accumulation, and fundus autofluorescence reveals a distinctive pattern. OCT provides adjunctive information regarding the location of the pathologic lesions with respect to the RPE, which can help confirm the diagnosis. In cases of known Stargardt disease, OCT is critical to detect and monitor macular atrophy that can develop parafoveally or subfoveally.

Key OCT Features

- There is disruption of the RPE and overlying outer retina and inner segment/outer segment/ellipsoid zone (IS/OS/EZ), which correlates with disease severity.
- Associated retinal atrophy begins in a parafoveal location (bulls-eye maculopathy), spreading to involve the fovea with longer disease duration (initially spares central fovea) (Figs. 26.2.2–26.2.4).

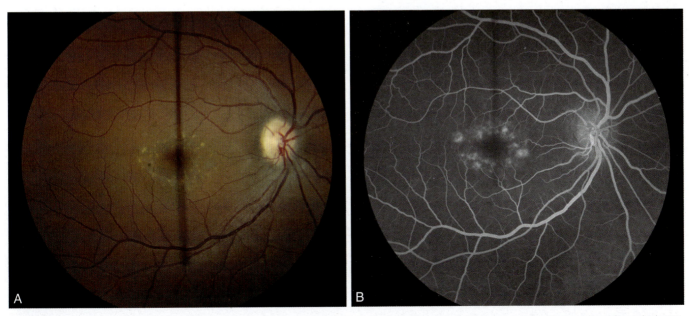

FIG. 26.2.1 (A) Color photograph of typical early Stargardt disease showing yellowish pisciform flecks. (B) Corresponding fluorescein angiograph shows staining of pisciform lesions and a characteristic dark choroid.

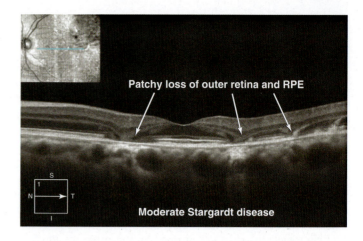

Patchy loss of outer retina and RPE

Moderate Stargardt disease

FIG. 26.2.3 Moderate Stargardt disease with patchy outer retinal and RPE atrophy. The central fovea is spared. *RPE*, Retinal pigment epithelium.

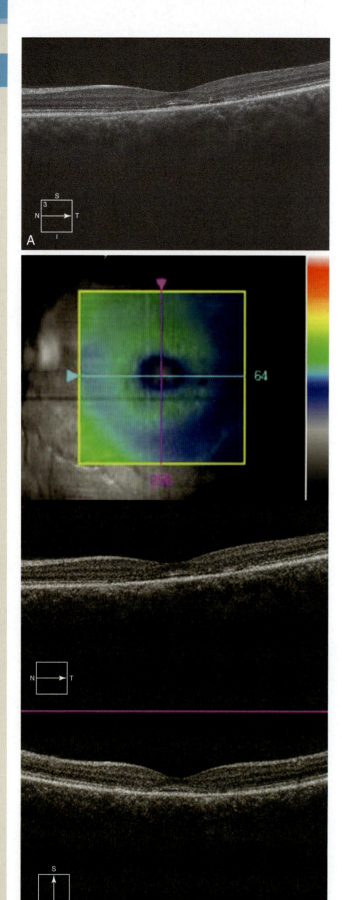

FIG. 26.2.2 (A) Structural OCT in mild Stargardt disease shows patchy disruption of the inner segment/outer segment/ellipsoid zone band in a parafoveal location. The central fovea is relatively intact. (B) Corresponding OCT thickness map reveals mild parafoveal thinning secondary to outer retinal loss.

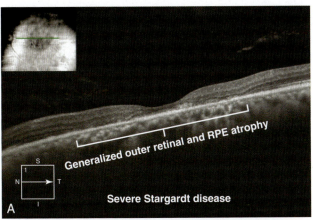

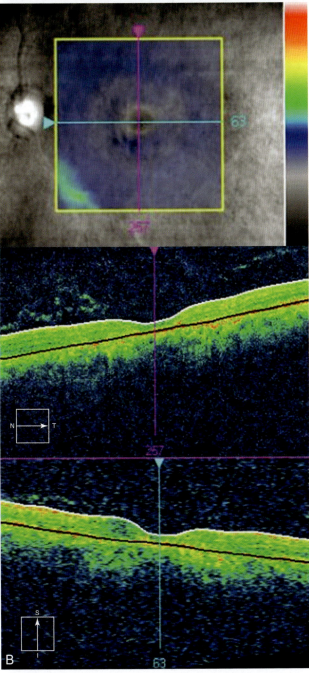

FIG. 26.2.4 (A) Structural OCT in severe/advanced Stargardt disease shows generalized outer retinal and RPE atrophy involving the entire macula. (B) Corresponding thickness map best illustrates the global macular atrophy. *RPE*, Retinal pigment epithelium.

Omar Abu-Qamar | Shilpa J. Desai*

Summary

Best disease or Best vitelliform macular dystrophy is an autosomal dominant genetic disorder caused by a mutation in the *BEST1* gene and features multiple clinical phenotypes during different stages of disease. These include the pre-vitelliform (abnormal electrooculogram [EOG]), vitelliform (egg-yolk lesion in fovea), pseudohypopyon, vitelleruptive (scrambled egg), and atrophic stages. The disease can be complicated by choroidal neovascularization in up to 20% of cases. Typically, there is a singular central macular lesion present bilaterally. However, multifocal and extrafoveal lesions can be seen in up to 30% of cases. OCT can identify representative submacular findings in Best disease, including differences among the various stages.

Key OCT Features

- Vitelliform stage exhibits thickening of the outer segment of photoreceptors and subretinal material that is a mix of both hyperreflective and hyporeflective material (Figs. 26.3.1–26.3.3).
- Pseudohypopyon stage exhibits layering of hyporeflective material superiorly and hyperreflective material inferiorly (layering of lipofuscin), which is best identified using a vertical OCT orientation (Figs. 26.3.4–26.3.6).
- Scrambled egg stage exhibits a mix of retinal pigment epithelium (RPE) atrophy, pigment clumping, and subretinal fibrosis.
- Atrophic stage exhibits generalized atrophy.

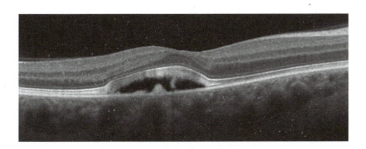

FIG. 26.3.1 Vitelliform stage of Best disease. Subretinal material is a mixture of hyperreflective and hyporeflective material.

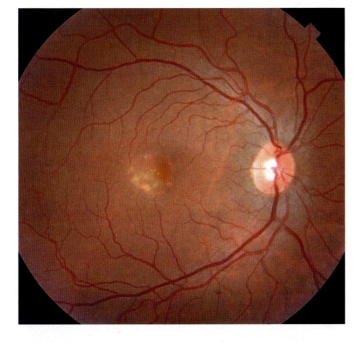

FIG. 26.3.2 Color photograph corresponding to Fig. 26.3.1.

*With contributions from Jay S. Duker

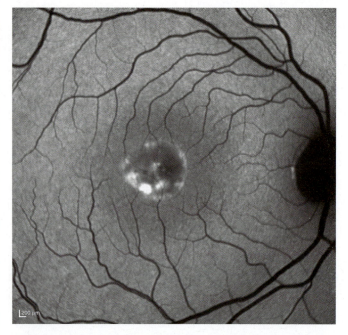

FIG. 26.3.3 Fundus autofluorescence corresponding to Fig. 26.3.1.

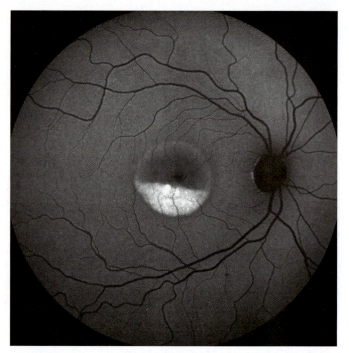

FIG. 26.3.6 Fundus autofluorescence corresponding to Fig. 26.3.4.

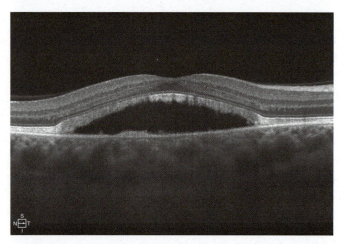

FIG. 26.3.4 Pseudohypopyon stage of Best disease, horizontal imaging plane through the superior component, which is hyporeflective.

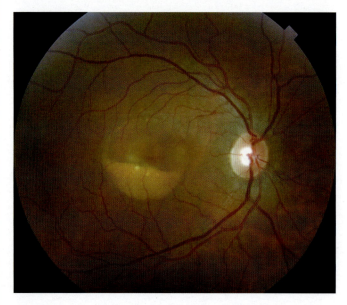

FIG. 26.3.5 Color photograph corresponding to Fig. 26.3.4.

Summary

Cone dystrophies encompass a number of heritable dystrophies affecting the cone system. As with other heritable conditions, the age of onset, severity, and rate of progression can vary depending on the mutation type. There have been several genes implicated in cone dystrophy (Renner et al., 2009). Symptoms include visual loss, impairment in color vision, and increased visual difficulty in brightly lit conditions (hemeralopia). Visual acuity is variable but typically ranges between 20/20 and 20/200. Fundus examination reveals a bull's-eye pattern of retinal pigment epithelium (RPE) atrophy within the macula, which is highlighted with fundus autofluorescence (Fig. 26.4.1). The peripheral retina is typically spared. OCT shows a loss of the outer retinal layers affecting the macula (Fig. 26.4.2). Electrophysiologic testing is often required to confirm the diagnosis and shows a decreased or undetectable photopic and flicker response.

Key Features

- Cone dystrophy refers to a wide variety of dystrophies characterized by dysfunction in the cone system.
- Clinical symptoms include loss of vision, impaired color vision, central scotoma, and hemeralopia.
- A bull's-eye maculopathy is the most characteristic clinical feature.
- OCT shows loss of the outer retinal layers affecting the macula and fovea, unlike in retinitis pigmentosa, in which there is often foveal sparing.
- OCT findings in advanced disease include complete atrophy of the macula.

REFERENCE

Renner, A. B., Fiebig, B. S., Weber, B. H., Wissinger, B., Andreasson, S., Gal, A., et al. (2009). Phenotypic variability and long-term follow-up of patients with known and novel PRPH2/RDS mutations. *American Journal of Ophthalmology*, *147*, 518–530.

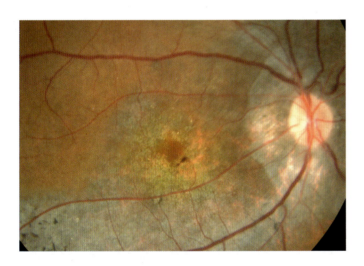

FIG. 26.4.1 Color fundus image showing retinal pigment epithelium loss at the fovea in a characteristic bulls eye pattern.

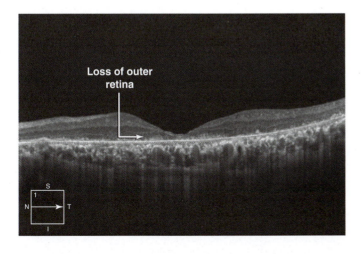

FIG. 26.4.2 OCT corresponding to Fig. 26.4.1. Line scan shows outer retinal loss through fovea and para-fovea.

Summary

Malattia leventinese, also referred to as familial dominant drusen, is caused by a known genetic defect (*EFEMP1*). The diagnosis is typically made based on the clinical appearance, which includes many variably sized, but predominantly large, drusen located within the central macula and peripapillary region, with smaller radially orientated drusen often seen temporal to the macula. The drusen appear at an early age compared to drusen resulting from age-related macular degeneration. Vision loss may occur because of the development of atrophic changes and secondary choroidal neovascularization. OCT is used predominantly as an adjuvant imaging modality to determine the extent and monitor the progression of secondary features of the disease.

Key OCT Features

- Focal dome-shaped, saw-tooth or diffuse hyperreflective deposits with retinal pigment epithelium elevations (i.e., drusen) between the retinal pigment epithelium and Bruch's membrane (Fig. 26.5.1).
- Small radial drusen, like cuticular drusen, may be present (Figs. 26.5.2–26.5.5).

BIBLIOGRAPHY

Querques, G., Guigui, B., Levezial, N., Querques, L., Bandello, F., & Souied, E. H. (2013). Multimodal morphological and functional characterization of malattia leventinese. *Graefe's Archive for Clinical and Experimental Ophthalmology*, 251(3), 705–714.

Zhang, T., Xie, X., Cao, G., Jiang, H., Wu, S., Su, Z., et al. (2014). Malattia leventinese/Doyne honeycomb retinal dystrophy in a Chinese family with mutation of the *EFEMP1* gene. *Retina*, 34(12), 2462–2471.

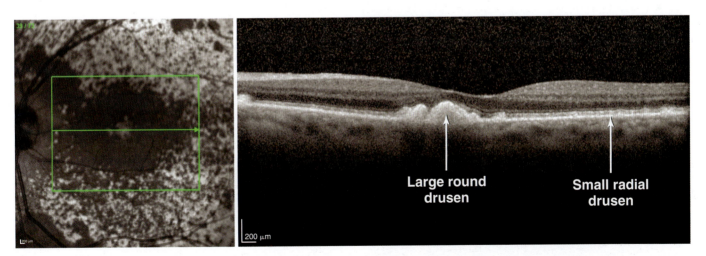

FIG. 26.5.1 OCT appearance of malattia leventinese with both large and small drusen.

*With contributions from Jay S. Duker

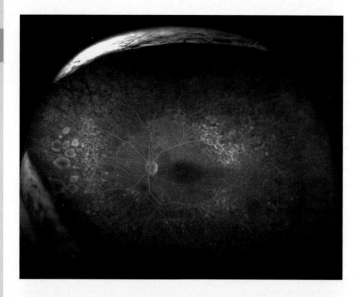

FIG. 26.5.2 Wide-field fluorescein angiogram corresponding to Fig. 26.5.1 illustrates the extent of peripheral drusen.

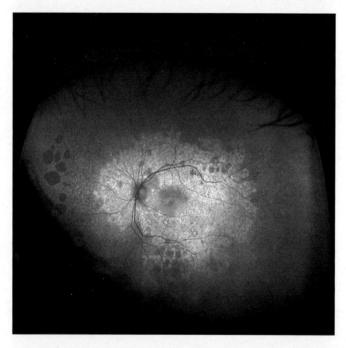

FIG. 26.5.3 Wide-field fundus autofluorescence demonstrates extensive peripheral retinal pigment epithelium dropout.

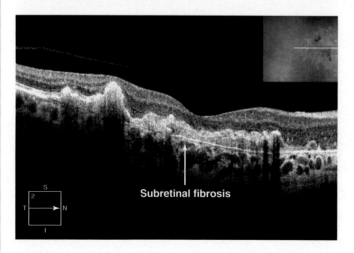

FIG. 26.5.4 Advanced malattia leventinese with subretinal fibrosis. (Courtesy Elias Reichel, MD.)

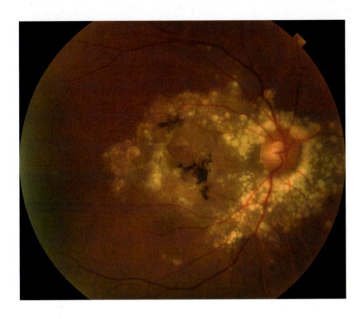

FIG. 26.5.5 Fundus photograph corresponding to Fig. 26.5.4 illustrates the classical appearance of malattia leventinese. (Courtesy Elias Reichel, MD.)

Central Areolar Choroidal Dystrophy

Jonathan T. Caranfa | Shilpa J. Desai*

26.6

Summary

Central areolar choroidal dystrophy (CACD) is an autosomal dominant inheritable disorder of the macula presenting between the second and fourth decades of life, with minimal focal parafoveal pigmentary changes. As the disease progresses poorly demarcated, round areas of hypopigmented atrophy develop with late stages of demonstrating well-defined atrophic areas with absence of retinal pigment epithelium (RPE), choriocapillaris, and neurosensory retina in the area of dystrophy exposing atrophic choroid (choroidal vessels can be seen coursing over bare sclera) (Boon et al., 2009).

Clinically, CACD can resemble age-related macular degeneration (AMD); however, patients with CACD are typically younger and have a strong family history of vision loss compared to those with AMD given the autosomal dominant inheritance pattern. OCT is useful to identify the key features of the disease at each stage and help distinguish this entity from AMD (Smailhodzic et al., 2011).

Key OCT Features

- The earliest features of disease include focal thickening and irregular reflectivity of the RPE that may resemble drusen.
- With moderate disease, outer retinal atrophic changes are present with an increase in distance between inner photoreceptor segments and photoreceptor outer segments/RPE band.
- In advanced stages of disease, generalized outer retinal, RPE, and choriocapillaris atrophy develop. An absence of sub-RPE deposits at this stage can help distinguish CACD from geographic atrophy secondary to AMD (Figs. 26.6.1 and 26.6.2).

REFERENCES

Boon, C. J. F., Klevering, B. J., Cremers, F. P. M., Zonneveld-Vrieling, M. N., Theelen, T., Den Hollander, A. I., et al. (2009). Central areolar choroidal dystrophy. *Ophthalmology, 116*(4), 771–782.

Smailhodzic, D., Fleckenstein, M., Theelen, T., Boon, C. J. F., van Huet, R. A. C., van de Ven, J. P. H., et al. (2011). Central areolar choroidal dystrophy (CACD) and age-related macular degeneration (AMD): Differentiating characteristics in multimodal imaging. *Investigative Ophthalmology & Visual Science, 52*(12), 8908–8918.

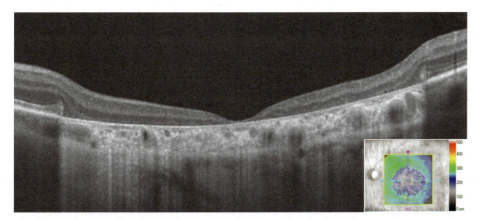

FIG. 26.6.1 OCT demonstrating advanced stage of central areolar choroidal dystrophy with atrophy of the outer retina, retinal pigment epithelium (RPE), and choriocapillaris. Note the absence of any sub-RPE deposits that would be more typical of geographic atrophy secondary to age-related macular degeneration.

*With contributions from Jay S. Duker

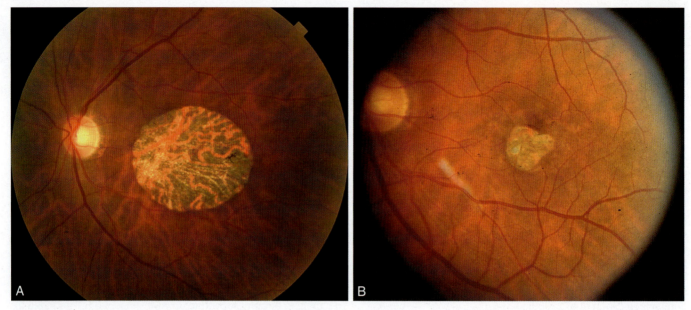

FIG. 26.6.2 (A) Fundus photograph showing well-demarcated area of chorioretinal atrophy, corresponding to Fig. 26.6.1. (B) Fundus photograph from the same patient 25 years earlier.

Stages of Posterior Vitreous Detachment

Darin R. Goldman

27.1

Summary

The vitreous is a dynamic substance that ages similarly to other parts of the body. This aging process results in ongoing liquefaction with weakening and eventual separation of vitreous adhesions to various structures in the posterior segment, including the optic nerve, macula, retinal blood vessels, and peripheral retina. The evolution of posterior vitreous detachment (PVD) occurs over many years through continuous vitreous separation from the posterior pole. The first stage of separation begins in the paramacular region (Fig 27.1.1 and 27.1.2) with eventual complete vitreopapillary separation. It is only this final event, which may take years to develop, that causes typical symptoms of an acute PVD with a visible Weiss ring clinically. Aberrant vitreous separation from posterior eye wall structures can result in a host of pathologic conditions such as vitreous hemorrhage, vitreomacular traction, macular hole, epiretinal membrane, retinal tear, and retinal detachment.

Key OCT Features

- Stages of PVD include *stage 1:* perifoveal PVD with intact vitreofoveal adhesion (Fig. 27.1.3); *stage 2:* isolated macular PVD with residual vitreopapillary adhesion (Fig. 27.1.4); *stage 3:* peripheral PVD with residual vitreopapillary adhesion (Fig. 27.1.5); *stage 4:* complete PVD (Fig. 27.1.6) (Johnson, 2005).
- Progressive stages (1–4) of PVD are all detectable via OCT (Fig. 27.1.7).

REFERENCE

Johnson, M. W. (2005). Perifoveal vitreous detachment and its macular complications. *Transactions of the American Ophthalmological Society, 103,* 537–567.

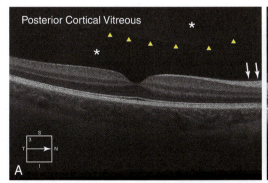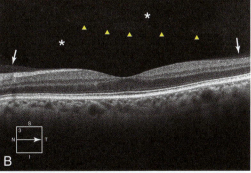

FIG. 27.1.1 OCT of a normal macula with attached posterior hyaloid. Although the vitreous cavity exhibits a generalized hyporeflective signal, the presence of attached posterior hyaloid (lack of a posterior vitreous detachment) is evident by a diffuse, faint, grainy lightly reflective signal *(asterisks).* Often, there will be a distinct demarcation *(arrowheads)* between layers of the posterior vitreous cortex that differ slightly in degree of reflectivity, which aids in confirmation of the presence of attached cortical vitreous. Additionally, the edges of the posterior hyaloid are visible as thin hyperreflective membranes *(arrows),* which blend almost imperceptibly with the surface of the macula. A and B distinguish R and L eyes, respectively.

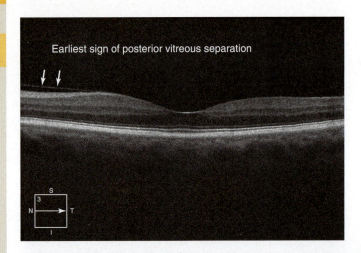

FIG. 27.1.2 The earliest sign of posterior vitreous separation is marked by focal separation between the posterior hyaloid and macular surface *(arrows)*.

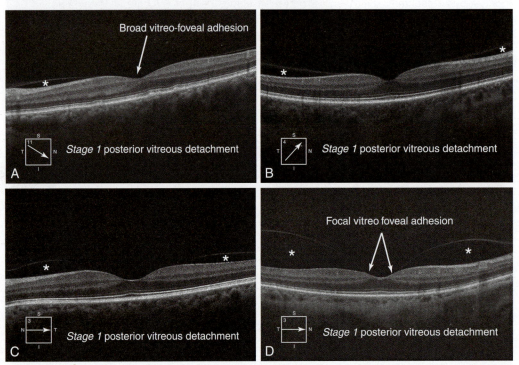

FIG. 27.1.3 Stage 1 posterior vitreous detachment is marked by posterior hyaloid separation from the surface of the retina surrounding the central fovea *(asterisks)*, while maintaining adhesions to the optic nerve and temporal to the macula. Within this stage, there is continued elevation of the hyaloid from a flat configuration (A and B) to one that is more bowed (C and D), and the area of foveal adhesion transitions from broad to more focal..

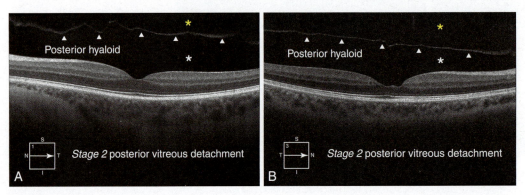

FIG. 27.1.4 Stage 2 posterior vitreous detachment results in complete release of vitreomacular attachment with residual adhesion to the temporal macula, optic nerve, and nasal periphery. At this stage, the posterior hyaloid face is easily visualized as a hyperreflective membrane above the macula *(arrowheads)*. The space between the posterior hyaloid and macula is generally darker or more hyporeflective *(white asterisk)* compared to the reflectivity of the vitreous *(yellow asterisk)*.

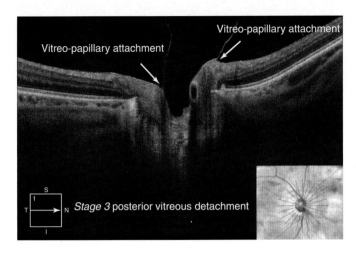

FIG. 27.1.5 OCT sectioned through the optic nerve head in stage 3 posterior vitreous detachment. There is residual vitreopapillary attachment *(arrows)*, and the posterior hyaloid has released from the entire retina anteriorly.

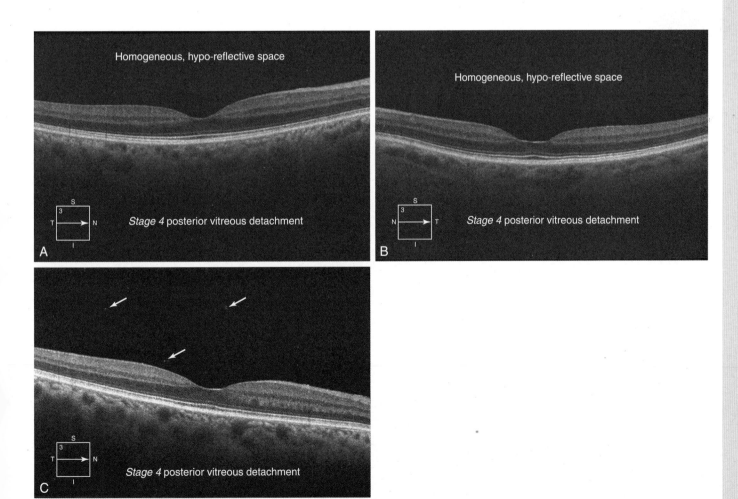

FIG. 27.1.6 Stage 4, or complete posterior vitreous detachment (PVD), is evident on OCT by a lack of any features of posterior vitreous that have been depicted in Figs. 27.1.1–27.1.3, 27.1.5, and 27.1.6. The vitreous cavity has a homogeneous, hyporeflective appearance. Secondary features associated with symptomatic stage 4 PVD, such as red blood cells in the setting of vitreous hemorrhage, may be visible (C, arrows).

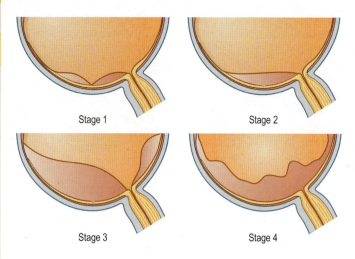

Stage 1

Stage 2

Stage 3

Stage 4

FIG. 27.1.7 Stages of PVD: *Stage 1* indicates perifoveal vitreous separation from the retina with intact vitreofoveal adhesion, *stage 2* indicates complete vitreous separation from the macula, *stage 3* indicates further separation of the vitreous from the peripheral retina while maintaining vitreopapillary adhesion, and *stage 4* indicates complete separation of the posterior vitreous from all attachments to the posterior segment. (From Johnson, M. W. (2005). Perifoveal vitreous detachment and its macular complications. Transactions of the American Ophthalmological Society 103, 537–567. Figure 2 [stages of PVD].)

Asteroid Hyalosis

Darin R. Goldman

Summary

Asteroid hyalosis is a benign condition resulting in vitreous opacities that appear as small, white, variably sized spheres ("stars in the night") dispersed throughout the vitreous cavity with a gravity-dependent distribution (Fig. 28.1.1A). The opacities generally produce no visual impairment for the patient; however, they can cause difficulty in clinical visualization and diagnosis of retinal abnormalities. The condition is unilateral or significantly greater in one than the other and occurs in approximately 1 in 100 people. In some cases in which asteroid hyalosis is dense and the macula cannot be viewed clinically, OCT can aid in visualizing macular detail and any associated macular pathologic processes (Fig. 28.1.1B). Asteroid hyalosis has a classic appearance on OCT as hyperreflective vertical streaks with varying widths.

Key OCT Features

- OCT is often able to visualize macular details even in the setting of severe asteroid hyalosis.
- Asteroid hyalosis spheres appear on OCT as hyperreflective vertically oriented streaks of varying width, which likely corresponds to the size of the sphere (Figs. 28.1.2–28.1.4).
- Although physically present only within the vitreous cavity, because of mirroring artifacts, lesions on OCT can appear to overlie the retinal layers and choroid.
- Shadowing effects are also characteristic of asteroid hyalosis and may be due to visualized flecks or those outside the frame of image capture.

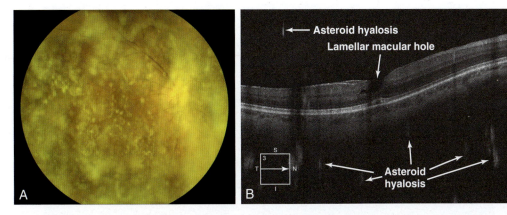

FIG. 28.1.1 (A) Color photograph of dense asteroid hyalosis, which obscures the ability to discern details of the underlying fundus. (B) Corresponding OCT has a reduced signal but reveals fairly good detail of the macula. In this particular case, there was concern for a possible full-thickness macular hole; however, OCT revealed a lamellar macular hole without full-thickness defect.

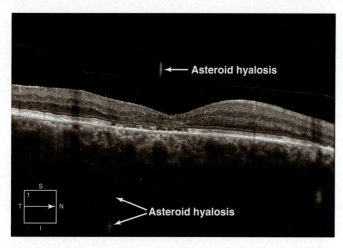

FIG. 28.1.2 Mild asteroid hyalosis with only a few lesions visible on OCT.

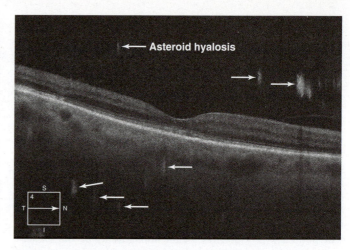

FIG. 28.1.3 Moderate asteroid hyalosis showing characteristic OCT appearance of hyperreflective, vertically oriented flecks *(arrows)*.

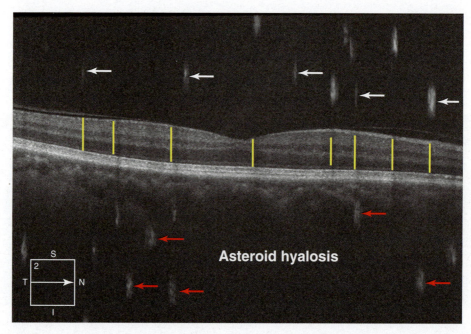

FIG. 28.1.4 Severe asteroid hyalosis showing many hyperreflective flecks. Note the numerous areas of shadowing artifact *(right side of yellow lines)*. These areas are associated with asteroid flecks located above *(white arrows, true image)* and below *(red arrows, mirrored artifact)* this plane.

Vitreous Hemorrhage

Darin R. Goldman

29.1

Summary

Spontaneous vitreous hemorrhage is a common disorder of the vitreous cavity, occurring in approximately 7 per 100,000 people (Spraul & Grossniklaus 1997). The appearance of vitreous hemorrhage develops secondary to bleeding from normal or neovascular blood vessels within the retina/vitreous and also may occur as a result of extension from layers underneath the retina. The most common causes for nontraumatic, spontaneous vitreous hemorrhage include diabetic retinopathy, retinal tear/detachment, vitreoretinal traction resulting from posterior vitreous detachment, retinal venous occlusive disease, ruptured retinal macroaneurysm, and exudative age-related macular degeneration. Spontaneous vitreous hemorrhage is a common cause for visual impairment and often will resolve without treatment in mild cases. More severe cases may require surgical vitrectomy. In the setting of severe vitreous hemorrhage and no visualization of the fundus, B-scan ultrasound is the imaging modality of choice. However, when vitreous hemorrhage is present with sufficient visualization of the fundus, OCT can be helpful to identify underlying macular abnormalities. Additionally, in cases of very subtle vitreous hemorrhage, OCT can be useful to confirm its presence.

Key OCT Features

- OCT findings in vitreous hemorrhage include visualization of individual red blood cells, clumps of hemorrhage, and secondary effects from shadowing (Figs. 29.1.1–29.1.4).
- Individual red blood cells appear as small, densely hyperreflective spots, whereas diffuse hemorrhage appears as a homogeneous sheet of hyperreflectivity.

REFERENCE

Spraul, C. W., & Grossniklaus, H. E. (1997). Vitreous hemorrhage. *Survey of Ophthalmology, 42*(1), 3–39.

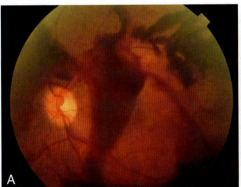
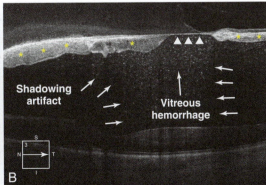

FIG. 29.1.1 (A) Color photograph of diabetic vitreous hemorrhage. (B) OCT visualizes the posterior hyaloid face *(arrowheads)* with underlying hemorrhage that is both attached to the back of the hyaloid *(asterisks)* and also dispersed within the underlying vitreous *(between arrows)*. Where the hemorrhage attached to the posterior hyaloid is thickest, the underlying details are obscured by shadowing artifact.

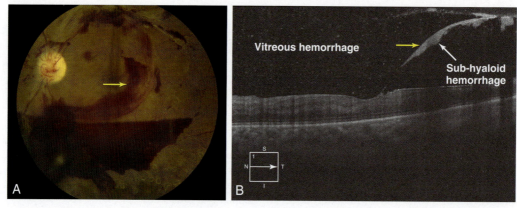

FIG. 29.1.2 (A) Color photograph of diabetic vitreous hemorrhage, mostly contained in the subhyaloid space. (B) OCT shows mild vitreous hemorrhage overlying the nasal macula. Temporally, there is subhyaloid hemorrhage (*yellow arrow* corresponds to same *arrow* in panel A) with underlying shadowing artifact.

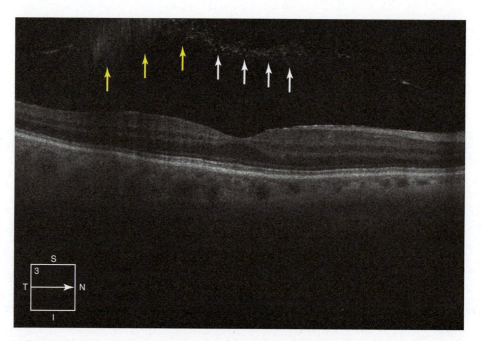

FIG. 29.1.3 Vitreous hemorrhage secondary to ruptured retinal macroaneurysm. Where the hemorrhage is denser, there is underlying shadowing artifact (*yellow arrows*). Where the hemorrhage is milder, there is no underlying shadowing (*white arrows*).

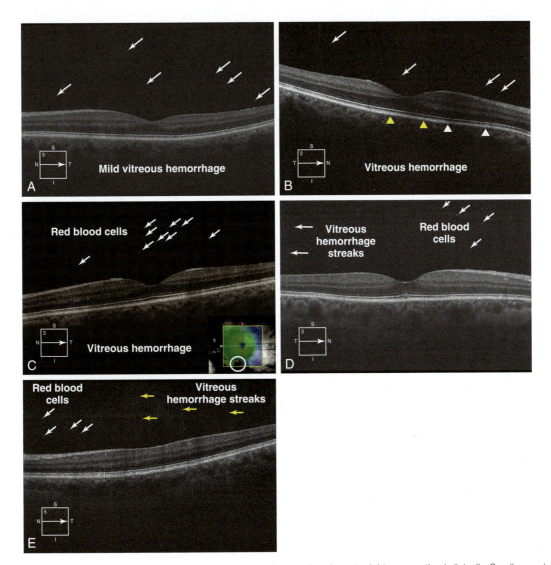

FIG. 29.1.4 (A) Mild vitreous hemorrhage in the setting of acute posterior vitreous detachment might go unnoticed clinically. Small, round, hyperreflective spots correspond to individual red blood cells *(arrows)*. (B) More significant vitreous hemorrhage with shadowing artifact *(between arrowheads)* from overlying vitreous hemorrhage, which is located above the imaged frame. Individual red blood cells are also visualized *(arrows)*. (C) In addition to red blood cells *(arrows)*, the thickness map reveals a black segmentation artifact *(circle)* that is due to localized signal blockage from overlying vitreous hemorrhage in this region. (D and E) Both red blood cells *(white arrows)* and hyperreflective, vertical streaks of vitreous hemorrhage *(yellow arrows)* are shown.

Vitreous Inflammation

Darin R. Goldman

30.1

Summary

A wide variety of uveitides result in vitreous inflammation as part of their disease course. The ability to monitor inflammation severity from visit to visit relies on an imprecise subjective clinical assessment that lacks reproducibility. OCT provides a more precise method to assess fluctuations in vitreous inflammation over time. The media opacity created by vitreous inflammation impairs transmission of light. The corresponding light attenuation is fairly evenly distributed and results in OCT signal degradation. In the absence of other causes for OCT signal loss, such as poor tear film or cataract, variation in OCT signal intensity can be useful in monitoring uveitis activity and response to treatment. The variation in OCT signal intensity, which correlates with vitritis severity, provides a direct measure of disease activity that is objective and reproducible (Figs. 30.1.1–30.1.3). Other, more sophisticated, methods for monitoring vitreous inflammation using OCT have been described (Keane et al., 2014; Zarranz-Ventura et al., 2016). Additionally, OCT is very useful to detect associated cystoid macular edema (CME) and monitor response to treatment *(arrows)*.

Key OCT Features

- OCT images acquired in the presence of vitreous inflammation will have loss of signal corresponding to the severity of vitreous opacity.
- OCT signal intensity can be used to monitor uveitis activity and response to treatment.
- Secondary effects of uveitis, such as CME, can be measured and monitored with precision in response to treatment.

REFERENCES

Keane, P. A., Karampelas, M., Sim, D. A., Sadda, S. R., Tufail, A., Sen, H. D., et al. (2014). Objective measurement of vitreous inflammation using optical coherence tomography. *Ophthalmology*, *121*(9), 1706–1714.

Zarranz-Ventura, J., Keane, P. A., Sim, D. A., Llorens, V., Tufail, A., Sadda, S. R., et al. (2016). Evaluation of objective vitritis grading method using optical coherence tomography: Influence of phakic status and previous vitrectomy. *American Journal of Ophthalmology*, *161*, 172–180.

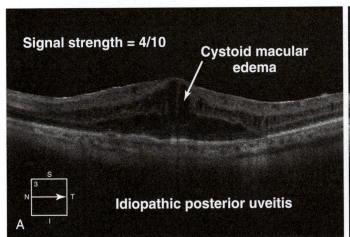
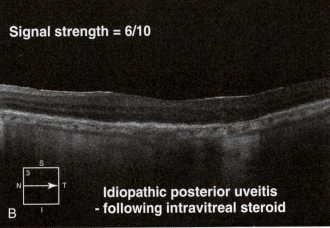

FIG. 30.1.1 (A) Idiopathic posterior uveitis. The signal strength is 4/10 because of diffuse vitreous inflammation, which is evidenced by the poor overall resolution of the image. There is also significant associated cystoid macular edema (CME). (B) At 1 month after intravitreal dexamethasone implant, CME resolved and signal strength improved to 6/10 along with improved vitreous inflammation. The improvements in signal strength and resolution of CME both indicate a positive response to treatment.

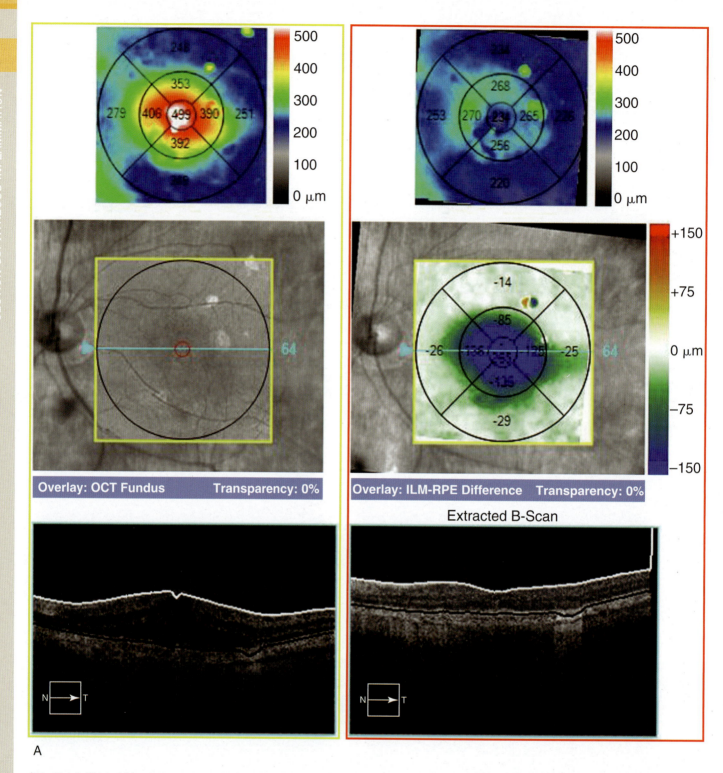

FIG. 30.1.2 (A) In addition to the structural OCT B-scan (*bottom*), thickness maps (*top*) and difference maps (*middle, right*) are very helpful in visualizing changes over time, particularly in response to treatment. Pretreatment (*yellow box*) thickness maps show significant central cystoid macular edema, which resolves after treatment (*red box*). This change over time is best visualized on the difference map (middle, right).

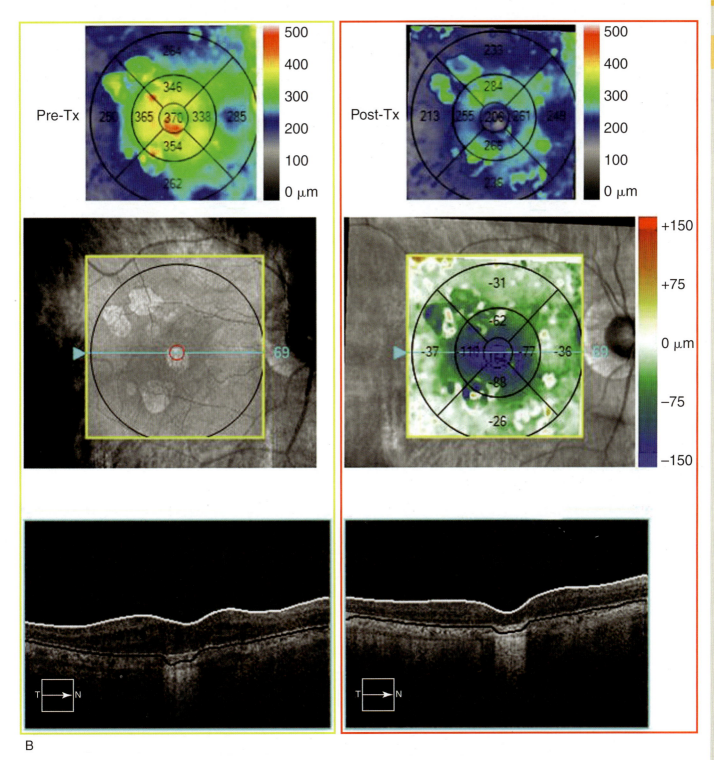

B

FIG. 30.1.2 cont'd. (B) A similar treatment response in the fellow eye is shown, highlighted by the thickness maps and difference map.

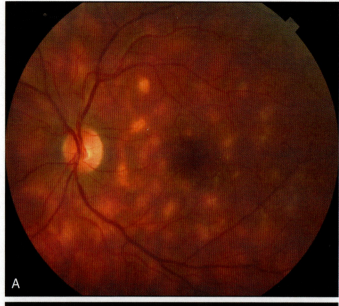

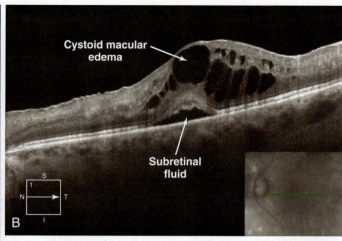

Cystoid macular edema

Subretinal fluid

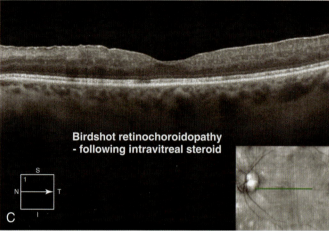

Birdshot retinochoroidopathy - following intravitreal steroid

FIG. 30.1.3 (A) Color photograph of birdshot retinochoroidopathy. (B) Pretreatment, there is significant cystoid macular edema (CME) and subretinal fluid. (C) After treatment with intravitreal steroid, there is complete resolution of CME and subretinal fluid.

Tractional Retinal Detachment

Darin R. Goldman

31.1

Summary

Tractional retinal detachment most commonly occurs secondary to proliferative diabetic retinopathy or proliferative vitreoretinopathy. The clinical appearance is characterized by visible epiretinal and vitreous membranes exerting tractional forces on the retinal surface. The type and location of retinal detachment depend on where these forces are applied and how strong they are. Isolated macular, isolated peripheral, or total retinal detachment can occur. The existence of a detachment is defined by the presence of subretinal fluid. Such fluid is often detectable on OCT before being visible clinically (Figs. 31.1.1–31.1.5). Tractional retinal detachments, in the setting of proliferative diabetic retinopathy, begin with focal traction on the retina, which progressively enlarges, causing thickening of the underlying retina with schisis-like changes and finally the development of underlying subretinal fluid. Tractional retinal detachments, in the setting of proliferative vitreoretinopathy, develop as a more acute process with prominent preretinal membranes and significant subretinal fluid.

Key OCT Features

- Tractional retinal detachments resulting from proliferative diabetic retinopathy are characterized by multifocal areas of traction, preretinal membranes, schisis-like changes within the retina, and areas of subretinal fluid (Figs. 31.1.1–31.1.4).
- Tractional retinal detachments secondary to other causes, such as proliferative vitreoretinopathy, have more prominent preretinal membranes and substantial amounts of subretinal fluid (Fig. 31.1.5).

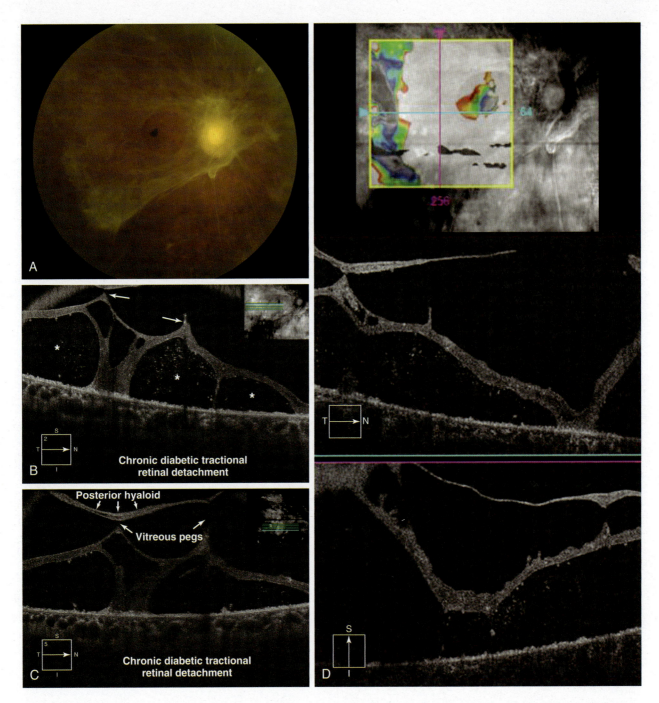

FIG. 31.1.1 (A) End-stage proliferative diabetic retinopathy with atrophic tractional retinal detachment in a "wolf-jaw" configuration. (B) OCT shows multiple areas of traction *(arrows)* and loculated subretinal fluid *(asterisks)*. The retina is severely attenuated and disorganized with loss of discernable layers. (C) The posterior hyaloid is visible with pegs of vitreous inserting onto the retinal surface. (D) OCT thickness map is limited because of segmentation errors, which are common in this setting.

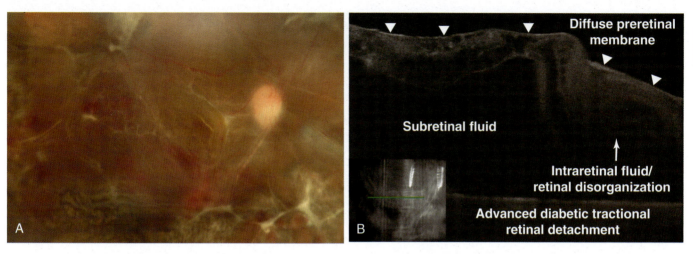

FIG. 31.1.2 (A) Advanced diabetic tractional retinal detachment involving the macula. (B) OCT reveals a diffuse membrane on the macular surface *(arrowheads)*, cystic intraretinal changes with retinal disorganization, a serpentine-like retinal arrangement, and significant subretinal fluid.

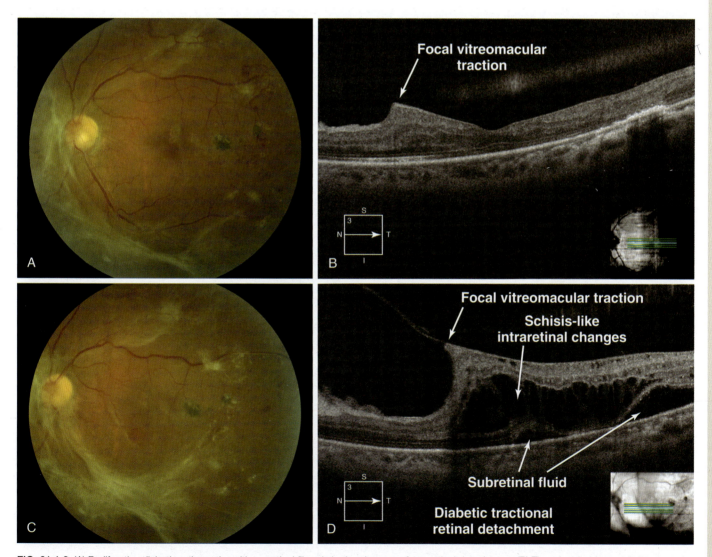

FIG. 31.1.3 (A) Proliferative diabetic retinopathy with preretinal fibrosis in the absence of any retinal detachment. (B) There is a focal area of vitreomacular traction but no detachment, because of the lack of subretinal fluid. (C) At a later date, the preretinal fibrovascular proliferation progressed to the point of causing a tractional retinal detachment involving the peripheral macula. (D) OCT reveals tractional separation of the retinal layers and subretinal fluid, which defines the presence of retinal detachment.

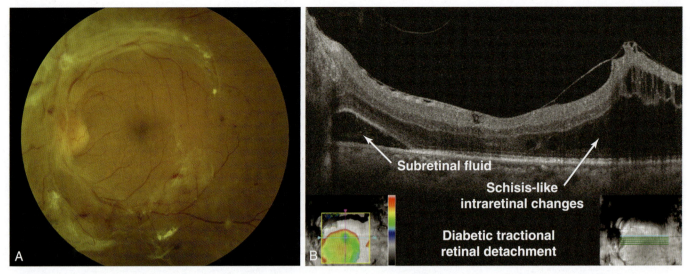

FIG. 31.1.4 (A) Diabetic tractional retinal detachment with early "wolf-jaw" configuration. (B) Structural OCT shows the presence of subretinal fluid nasal to the fovea and tractional thickening, or schisis-like changes, temporal to the fovea. The OCT thickness map (*inset, bottom-left*) is useful to better illustrate the three-dimensional nature of the tractional effect exerted in a circumferential manner on the edges of the macula.

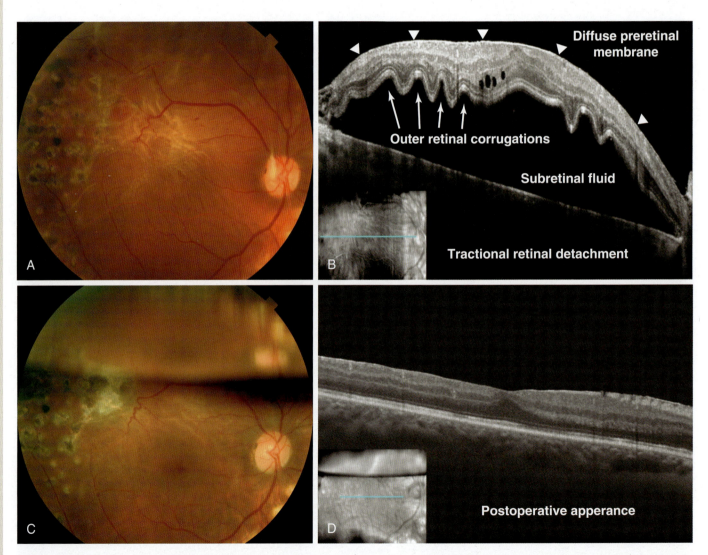

FIG. 31.1.5 (A) Tractional retinal detachment secondary to proliferative vitreoretinopathy after unsuccessful primary rhegmatogenous retinal detachment repair. (B) There is a thick, diffuse preretinal membrane along the surface of the macula (*arrowheads*) that gives the macular surface a smooth appearance. Additionally, there is significant underlying subretinal fluid and a corrugated configuration to the outer retinal surface (*arrows*). (C) After surgical repair, the preretinal membranes have been removed, and the macula is reattached. A residual intravitreal gas bubble is visible superiorly. (D) OCT shows complete resolution of the preretinal membrane with a smooth macular contour and no subretinal fluid.

Rhegmatogenous Retinal Detachment | 31.2

Darin R. Goldman

Summary

Rhegmatogenous retinal detachment (RRD) results from subretinal fluid accumulation underneath the retina after a retinal break. The detachment starves the retina of nourishment, with resultant damage to photoreceptors over time. If the central macula is involved, vision loss occurs that recovers to a variable degree after successful reattachment. This visual recovery correlates best with presenting visual acuity but has proved difficult to predict. However, OCT may provide insight into predicting and monitoring visual recovery based on identifiable anatomic changes. Although these anatomic alterations are not well understood, both qualitative and quantitative changes within the photoreceptor microstructure are thought to be largely responsible. Various studies have attempted to clarify these suspicions using primarily OCT-based end points. OCT findings have been shown to correlate with final visual acuity after macula-involving retinal detachments, including outer nuclear layer thinning and ellipsoid zone irregularities (Sridhar & Flynn, 2014). Additionally, overall photoreceptor thickness may correlate with visual recovery after retinal reattachment with an initial thinning followed by normalization, which coincides with visual recovery (Terauchi et al., 2015). Another potentially useful parameter measurable on OCT is the optical density of subretinal fluid, which increases with duration of detachment and correlates with postoperative visual acuity (Leshno et al., 2015).

Key OCT Features

- Subretinal fluid is present, evidenced by a homogeneous hyporeflective space underneath the neurosensory retina, which increases in height from nasal to temporal (Figs. 31.2.1–31.2.8).
- The underlying retinal pigment epithelium (RPE) remains attached with a smooth contour, which can be visualized in shallow detachments.
- In acute detachments, retinal corrugations and cystoid edema are present (Fig. 31.2.1).
- In chronic detachments, a relatively flat configuration and atrophic retinal changes are seen (Figs. 31.2.6 and 31.2.8).
- Microstructural changes within the photoreceptor layers correlate with final visual acuity.
- Optical density of subretinal fluid increases with duration of detachment.
- The most useful OCT output formats to determine whether subretinal fluid involves the fovea are thickness maps and vertically oriented B-scans.

REFERENCES

Leshno, A., Barak, A., Loewenstein, A., Weinberg, A., & Neudorfer, M. (2015). Optical density of subretinal fluid in retinal detachment. *Investigative Ophthalmology & Visual Science, 56*(9), 5432–5438.

Sridhar, J., & Flynn, H. W., Jr. (2014). Spectral-domain optical coherence tomography imaging of macula-off rhegmatogenous retinal detachment. *Clinical Ophthalmology, 8,* 561–566.

Terauchi, G., Shinoda, K., Matsumoto, C. S., Watanabe, E., Matsumoto, H., & Mizota, A. (2015). Recovery of photoreceptor inner and outer segment layer thickness after reattachment of rhegmatogenous retinal detachment. *British Journal of Ophthalmology, 99*(10), 1323–1327.

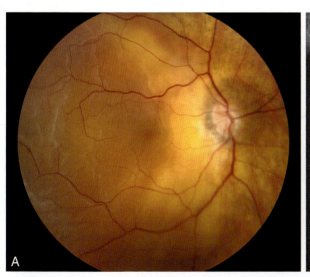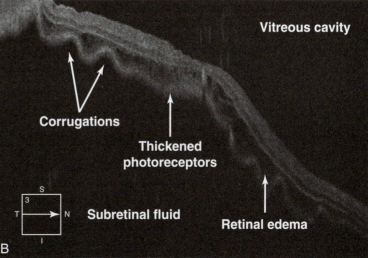

FIG. 31.2.1 (A) Color photograph of a macula-off rhegmatogenous retinal detachment within 2 weeks of symptom onset. (B) OCT shows corrugations of the underlying retinal surface, diffuse retinal edema, and enlargement of the photoreceptors.

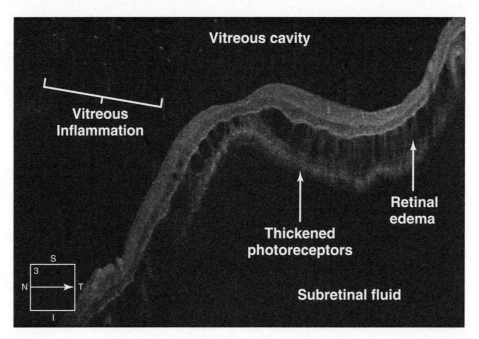

FIG. 31.2.2 Macula-off rhegmatogenous detachment illustrates retinal edema, thickened photoreceptors, and vitreous inflammation, which suggests a longer duration of detachment.

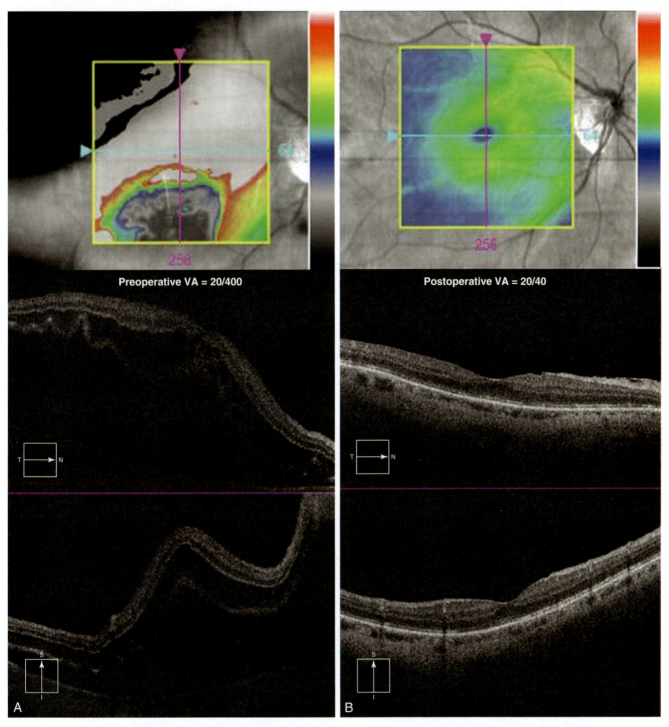

Preoperative VA = 20/400

Postoperative VA = 20/40

FIG. 31.2.3 (A) Preoperative OCT of macula-off rhegmatogenous retinal detachment with visual acuity of 20/400. (B) Postoperative OCT 1 month after reattachment of the retina by vitrectomy. Visual acuity (*VA*) improved to 20/40. On reattachment, resolution of subretinal fluid, retinal edema, and retinal corrugations are seen, with restoration of a fairly normal macular contour. The retinal thickness, mostly the result of photoreceptor integrity, remains normal.

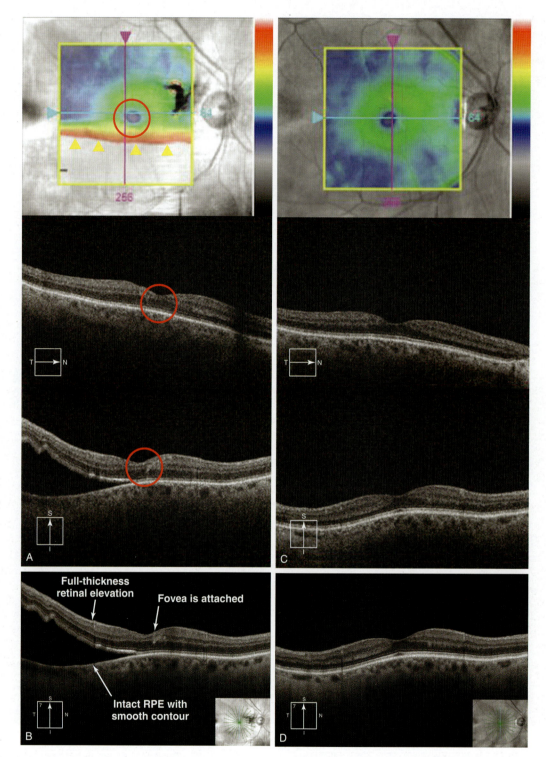

FIG. 31.2.4 Macula-involving, but fovea-on, rhegmatogenous retinal detachment. (A) Thickness map *(top)* illustrates the border of the detached retina *(yellow arrowheads)*, located inferior to the fovea. The fovea remains attached *(circles)*. (B) Vertically oriented B-scan image best illustrates the extent of the subretinal fluid and is useful to evaluate the status of the fovea. (C and D) At 6 months after surgical reattachment, the macula has regained a normal appearance, and the fovea is completely reattached.

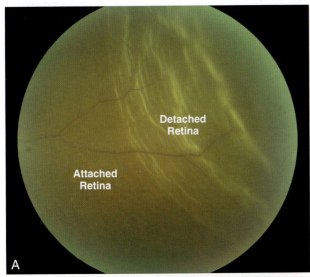

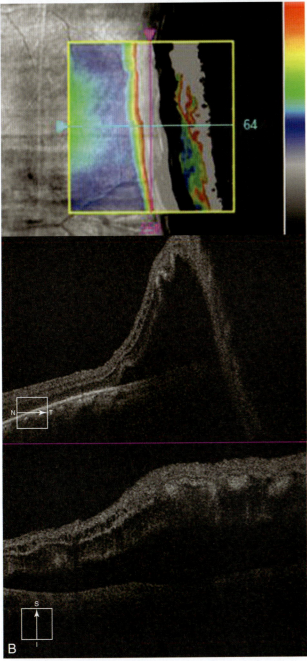

FIG. 31.2.5 Rhegmatogenous retinal detachment secondary to giant retinal tear. (A) Color photograph illustrates attached and detached retina. (B) Corresponding OCT at the border between attached and detached retina.

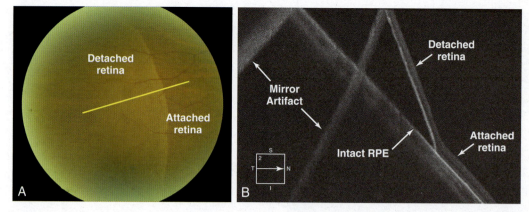

FIG. 31.2.6 Chronic rhegmatogenous retinal detachment. (A) Color photograph illustrates the absence of retinal corrugations. (B) Corresponding OCT (*line* in color photograph indicates cross-section) shows distinct areas of attached and detached retina. The detached retina is flat and somewhat attenuated. Note the dual mirror artifacts with inverted images. *RPE*, Retinal pigment epithelium.

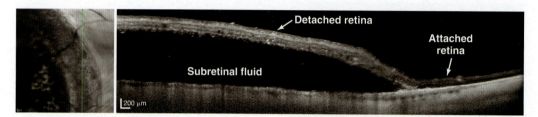

FIG. 31.2.7 The transition zone from attached retina to detached retina is illustrated. (Courtesy Netan Choudhry, MD.)

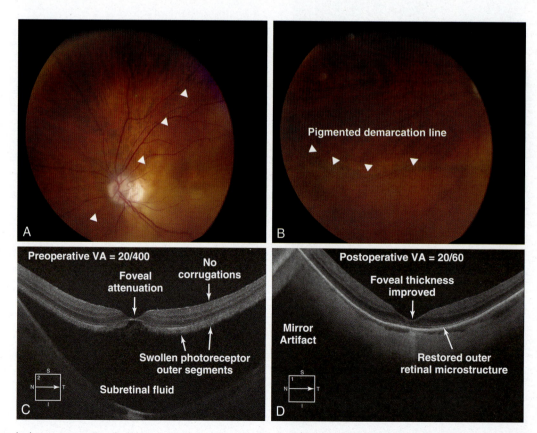

FIG. 31.2.8 Chronic rhegmatogenous retinal detachment with presenting visual acuity *(VA)* of 20/400. (A) Color photograph centered on the optic nerve shows subretinal fluid in the macula (within *arrowheads*). (B) Color photograph of the inferonasal periphery reveals a pigmented demarcation line, indicative of chronicity. (C) Preoperative OCT through the fovea shows a smooth contour of the retina with significant subretinal fluid. The central fovea is attenuated, and the photoreceptor outer segments are markedly swollen. (D) At 3 months after surgical reattachment of the retina, the foveal thickness increased to near normal and the outer retinal bands are restored. VA returned to 20/60. Note the presence of a myopic staphyloma.

Bullous Retinoschisis

Darin R. Goldman

31.3

Summary

Bullous senile retinoschisis involves splitting of the retina along a plane within or between a particular retinal layer or layers. Although schisis is most commonly located in the superotemporal peripheral retina, it may occur in any meridian and is often bilateral. Schisis is typically limited to the peripheral retina but may communicate posteriorly and involve the macula. The involved retina appears smoothly elevated, which may be difficult to distinguish from rhegmatogenous retinal detachments. This distinction is critical to avoid unnecessary intervention in the case of retinoschisis and guide appropriate treatment in the case of retinal detachment. Certain clinical signs and diagnostic evaluation, such as visual field testing or laser demarcation, can help clarify the diagnosis, although these methods are not definitive. OCT provides an unequivocal method of distinguishing retinoschisis from retinal detachment (Figs. 31.3.1–31.3.7). Multiple, separate areas of the retina should be imaged to increase the likelihood of identifying any associated detachment that could be overlooked by imaging only one location. Because of the typical peripheral location of retinoschisis, OCT imaging can be cumbersome and therefore may be underutilized. Orientation of the OCT imaging plane perpendicular to the elevated area while including the retinal transition from flat to elevated is helpful.

Key OCT Features

- OCT provides a definitive method of differentiating retinal elevations resulting from retinoschisis or retinal detachment (Figs. 31.3.1–31.3.7).
- Schisis is defined by a separation within the retina that occurs between the inner and outer retinal layers, always leaving outer retinal layers (ORLs) overlying the retinal pigment epithelium (RPE). This is in contrast to retinal detachment, in which the plane of separation is between the RPE and neurosensory retina.
- At least two distinct partitions of split retina are visible with intervening connecting strands of stretched retinal elements, thought to be Müller's cells.
- Retinal separation widens from posterior to anterior.

BIBLIOGRAPHY

Choudhry, N., Golding, J., Manry, M. W., & Rao, R. C. (2016). Ultra-widefield steering-based spectral domain optical coherence tomography imaging of the retinal periphery. *Ophthalmology, 123*(6), 1368–1374.

Stehouwer, M., Tan, S. H., van Leeuwen, T. G., & Verbraak, D. L. (2014). Senile retinoschisis versus retinal detachment, the additional value of peripheral retinal OCT scans (SLSCAN-1, Topcon). *Acta Ophthalmologica, 92*(3), 221–227.

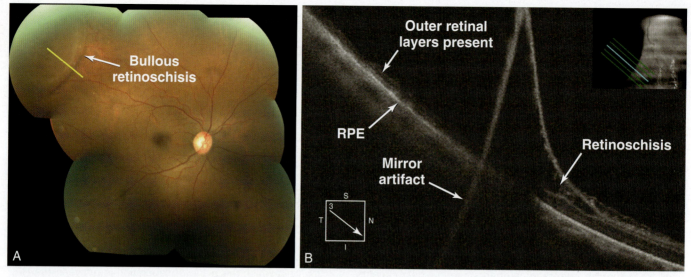

FIG. 31.3.1 (A) Color photograph of bullous retinoschisis located in the superotemporal retinal periphery. (B) OCT obtained with the scanning plane orthogonal to elevated retina, while still including a portion of flat retina (see *yellow line*, panel A). Note that in the area where the retina is most elevated, outer retinal layers are visible overlying the RPE, which defines schisis on OCT. *RPE*, Retinal pigment epithelium.

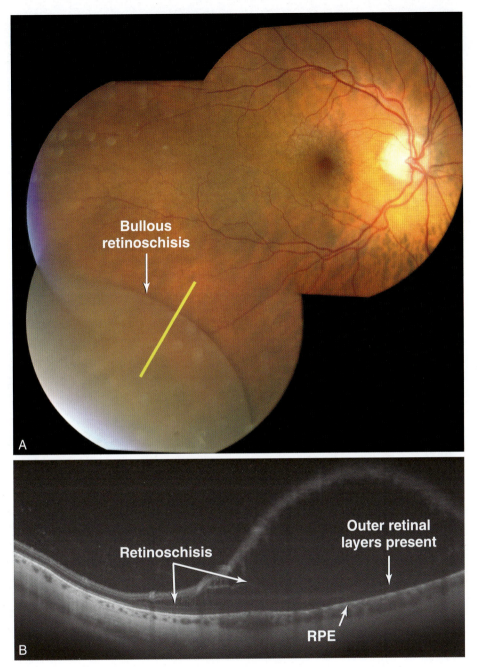

FIG. 31.3.2 (A) Color photograph of bullous retinoschisis located in the inferotemporal retinal periphery. (B) OCT was obtained with the scanning plane orthogonal to the elevated retina, while still including a portion of flat retina (see *yellow line*, panel A). ORLs are visible overlying the RPE, which defines schisis on OCT. *RPE*, Retinal pigment epithelium.

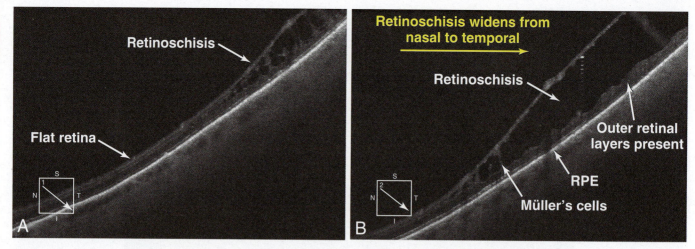

FIG. 31.3.3 (A) Transition zone from flat retina to shallow retinoschisis is illustrated. (B) More of the area of retinoschisis is shown, which widens from left to right (nasal to temporal). Connecting elements, thought to be Müller's cells, are visible, and outer retinal layers are present overlying the RPE. *RPE*, Retinal pigment epithelium.

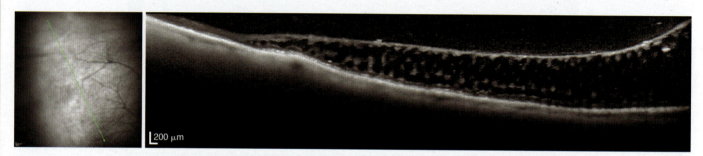

FIG. 31.3.4 Shallow retinoschisis with interweaving retinal elements that appear stretched. (Courtesy Netan Choudhry, MD.)

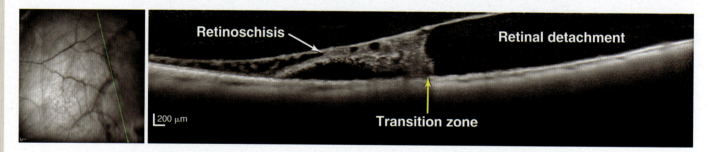

FIG. 31.3.5 Combined retinoschisis and retinal detachment. Both areas are distinctly visualized on each side of the transition zone *(yellow arrow)*. (Courtesy Netan Choudhry, MD.)

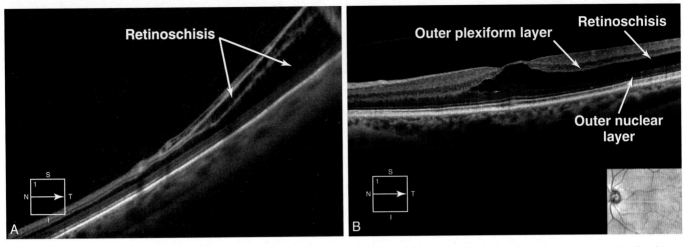

FIG. 31.3.6 (A) Peripheral retinoschisis includes multiple planes of separation. (B) The peripheral retinoschisis communicates posteriorly to involve the macula, where the plane of separation is easier to determine between the outer plexiform layer and outer nuclear layers.

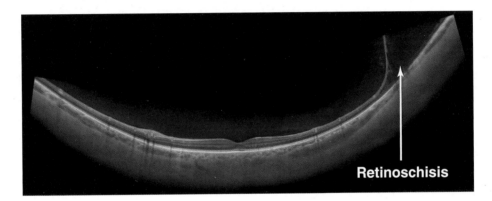

FIG. 31.3.7 Wide-angle OCT imaging the retina from ora to ora. Bullous retinoschisis is visible temporally. (Courtesy Netan Choudhry, MD.)

Summary

Lattice degeneration is a common retinal disorder that affects the peripheral retina and increases the risk for developing a retinal tear or retinal detachment. Lattice degeneration is present to some degree in 5% to 10% of the population, varies in extensiveness, and is usually asymptomatic. The presence of lattice degeneration is typically detected as an incidental finding during routine ophthalmoscopy. The clinical appearance can vary widely but generally includes thin, well-demarcated, pigmented ovoid patches of retina located in a circumferential orientation. Within the involved area, there may be sclerotic vessels or atrophic holes. Although usually darkly pigmented, lattice degeneration may appear hypopigmented (Fig. 31.4.1). The vitreous overlying lattice degeneration is liquefied, and, on the edges of lattice, there is firm vitreoretinal adhesion, which has been established mostly by histopathologic studies. The vitreoretinal interface has not been well studied using OCT, although OCT provides a unique opportunity to evaluate this entity in vivo. The difficulty in imaging lattice degeneration with OCT is due to its peripheral location. This can be overcome with a skilled photographer and cooperative patient. In the future, OCT imaging modalities may include modifications that assist with peripheral imaging, which would make its use more practical for lattice degeneration.

Key OCT Features

- Lattice degeneration is characterized by firm vitreoretinal adhesions on the edges with clear vitreous overlying the lesion.
- The involved retina typically demonstrates generalized thinning (Figs. 31.4.2–31.4.7).
- Subclinical retinal detachment is very common, a feature best appreciated on OCT (Figs. 31.4.4–31.4.7).
- U-shaped (in cross-section) overlying vitreous insertion/traction is common (Fig. 31.4.4).

BIBLIOGRAPHY

Manjunath, V., Taha, M., Fujimoto, J. G., & Duker, J. S. (2011). Posterior lattice degeneration characterized by spectral domain optical coherence tomography. *Retina*, *31*(3), 492–496.

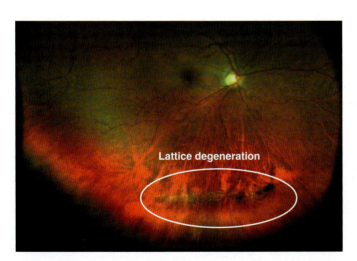

FIG. 31.4.1 Wide-field image illustrating characteristic appearance of lattice degeneration. (Courtesy Netan Choudhry, MD.)

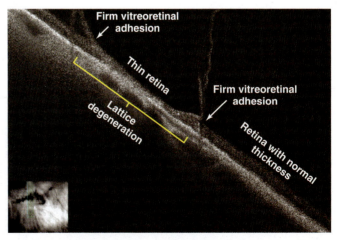

FIG. 31.4.2 The OCT imaging plane is oriented perpendicular to the short axis of lattice degeneration. The involved retina is thin, with firm vitreoretinal adhesion to both edges of the lattice degeneration.

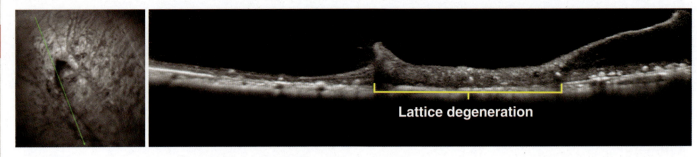

FIG. 31.4.3 In this example of lattice degeneration, there is broad vitreoretinal traction over the involved region that creates an appearance of localized retinal thickening. (Courtesy Netan Choudhry, MD.)

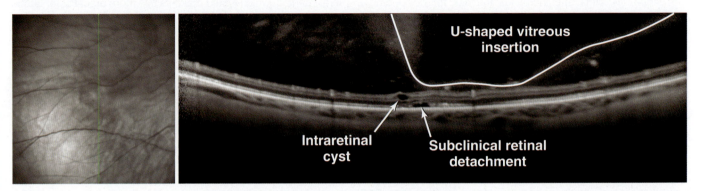

FIG. 31.4.4 The area imaged is just on the edge of a small area of lattice degeneration, which highlights the abnormal appearance of the overlying vitreous. The vitreous is thickened, appearing as a broad, U-shaped, hyperreflective band *(white line)*. Secondary features, including a small subclinical retinal detachment and an intraretinal cyst, are also visible. (Courtesy Netan Choudhry, MD.)

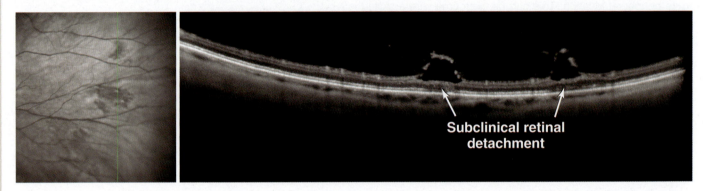

FIG. 31.4.5 Two small areas of lattice degeneration are shown that have an atypical OCT appearance. The focal vitreoretinal traction overlying each area has created a schisis-like effect. Splitting and elevation of the inner retinal layers are seen toward the vitreous cavity. (Courtesy Netan Choudhry, MD.)

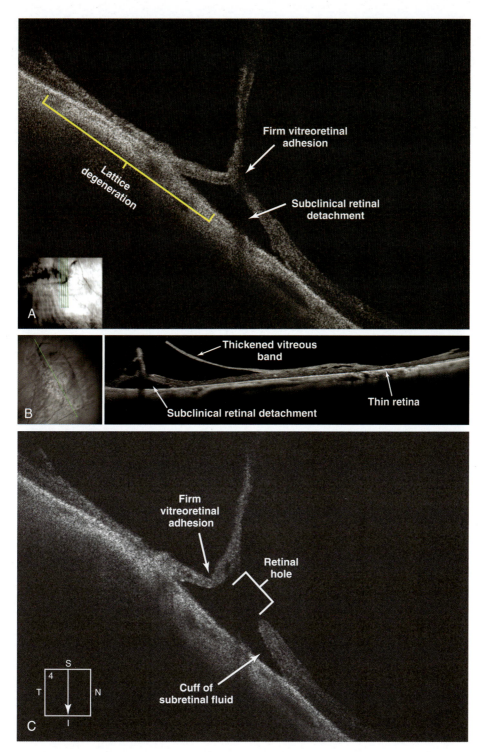

FIG. 31.4.6 (A) At the edge of this area of lattice degeneration, there is firm vitreoretinal adhesion causing a subclinical retinal detachment, which was not visible clinically. (B) Many of the features of lattice degeneration visible on OCT are illustrated. (C) A retinal break is present at the edge of vitreoretinal traction, along with a small cuff of subclinical subretinal fluid. (Panel B courtesy Netan Choudhry, MD.)

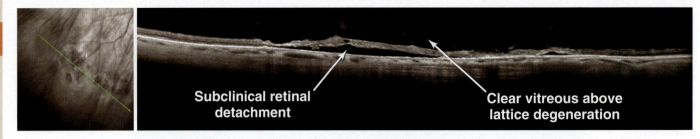

FIG. 31.4.7 A subclinical retinal detachment is shown, associated with typical lattice degeneration. The vitreous immediately overlying the lattice degeneration is optically empty and completely hyporeflective compared to the surrounding vitreous, which exhibits some degree of granular reflectivity. (Courtesy Netan Choudhry, MD.)

Myelinated Nerve Fiber Layer

Darin R. Goldman

31.5

Summary

Myelinated nerve fiber layer (mNFL) is a benign clinical entity that results from an embryologic developmental anomaly, whereby focal areas of the retinal nerve fiber layer fail to lose their myelin sheath. Clinically, mNFL appears as distinct white patches on the inner retinal surface. This appearance may mimic acute pathologic retinal conditions such as retinal edema from branch retinal artery occlusion, acute retinal necrosis, or retinal vasculitis. Given the benign nature of mNFL, the distinction is crucial. OCT exhibits characteristic features that are helpful to confirm the diagnosis of mNFL (Figs. 31.5.1–31.5.3). These features include a homogeneous, highly reflective band in the affected area of the retina that is isolated to the most superficial retinal layer. Areas of mNFL vary in thickness but are thickest toward their center. The associated intense hyperreflectivity results in underlying shadowing. This shadowing causes a loss of the distinction to the outer retinal layers, the degree of which correlates with the thickness of the mNFL. Blood vessels within the mNFL are highlighted by the contrast in reflectivity between the adjacent mNFL and relatively hyporeflective vessel lumen. In distinction to other, similar-appearing pathologic entities, there is no associated cystoid macular edema, retinal atrophy, overlying vitreous inflammation, or dynamic changes over time.

Key OCT Features

- The mNFL displays characteristic OCT features, including extreme hyperreflectivity of the involved superficial retinal layer with underlying shadowing that correlates with the thickness of the mNFL.
- There is absence of any associated retinal thinning or overlying vitreous inflammation.
- The OCT appearance remains stable over time.

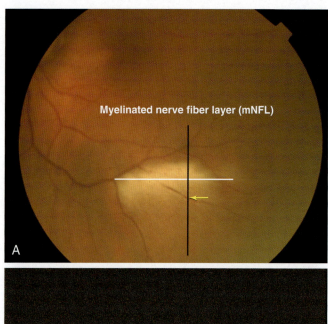

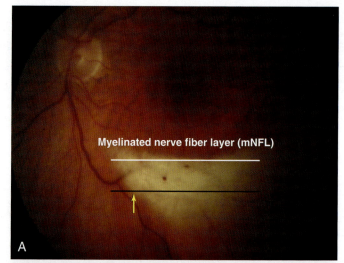

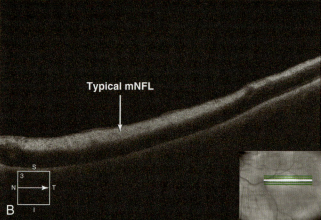

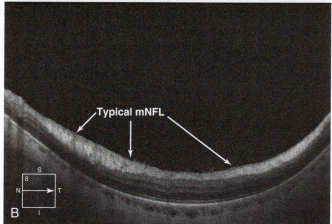

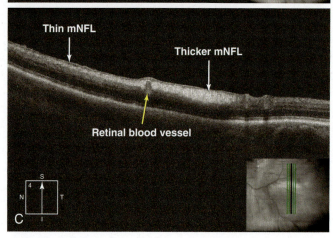

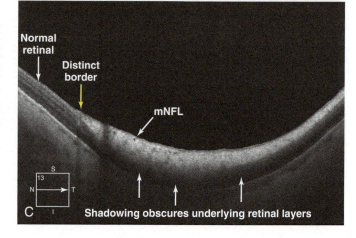

FIG. 31.5.1 (A) Color photograph of typical mNFL. The inner retina is involved with some obscuration of retinal blood vessels. (B) Horizontal OCT imaging plane illustrates characteristic intense, diffuse hyperreflectivity of the involved region on the inner retinal surface. The underlying retinal layers are not discernable because of shadowing. (C) Vertical OCT imaging plane transects both thinner and thicker regions of the mNFL. In the thin area, underlying retinal layers are discernable, whereas in the thicker area, underlying retinal layers are obscured by shadowing. Note the blood vessel that is highly visible within the mNFL because of the contrasting reflectivity of the mNFL and vessel lumen (*yellow arrow* in A and C). *mNFL,* Myelinated nerve fiber layer.

FIG. 31.5.2 (A) Color photograph of the mNFL located on the inferior edge of the macula. (B) Horizontally oriented OCT image toward superior edge of the mNFL (plane corresponds to *white line* in A), which captures both thin and thick areas of the mNFL with varying degrees of underlying shadowing, which correlates to the thickness of the mNFL. Characteristic extreme, diffuse hyperreflectivity of the mNFL is present. (C) Horizontally oriented OCT image within the midsection of the mNFL (plane corresponds to *black line* in A). Because of the thickness of the mNFL in this region, the underlying retina is obscured from significant shadowing. Note that the border between normal retina and mNFL is distinct (*yellow arrow* in A and C). *mNFL,* Myelinated nerve fiber layer.

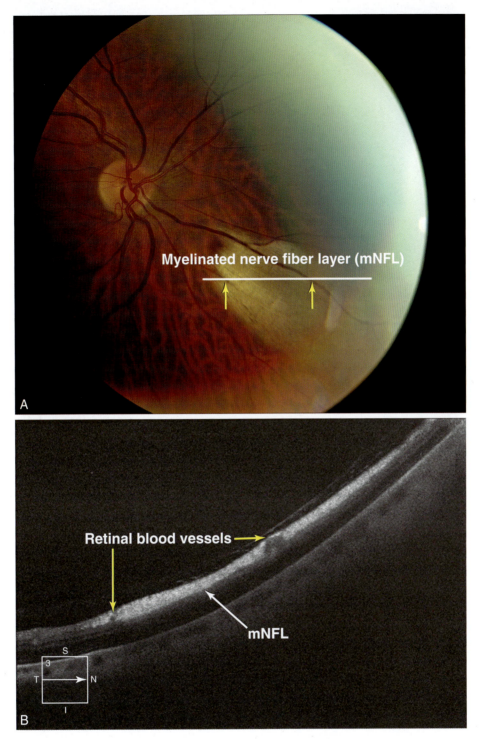

FIG. 31.5.3 (A) Color photograph of mNFL located inferonasally. (B) OCT through mNFL and two interspersed retinal blood vessels. *mNFL*, Myelinated nerve fiber layer.

Index

Page numbers followed by "*f*" indicate figures.

W

X